MILADY'S STANDARD
Professional Barbering
Student Workbook

Maura Scali-Sheahan, Ed.D.

Australia • Brazil • Japan • Korea • Mexico • Singapore • Spain • United Kingdom • United States

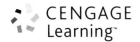
CENGAGE
Learning™

MILADY'S STANDARD Professional Barbering Student Workbook, Fifth Edition
Maura Scali-Sheahan, Ed.D.

President, Milady: Dawn Gerrain

Publisher: Erin O'Connor

Acquisitions Editor: Martine Edwards

Product Manager: Jessica Mahoney

Editorial Assistant: Maria Hebert

Director of Beauty Industry Relations:
Sandra Bruce

Senior Marketing Manager: Gerard McAvey

Production Director: Wendy Troeger

Senior Content Project Manager:
Nina Tucciarelli

Senior Art Director: Joy Kocsis

For product information and technology assistance, contact us at
Professional & Career Group Customer Support, 1-800-648-7450

For permission to use material from this text or product,
submit all requests online at **cengage.com/permissions.**
Further permissions questions can be emailed to
permissionrequest@cengage.com.

Library of Congress Control Number: 2010904304

ISBN-13: 978-1-4354-9713-9

ISBN-10: 1-4354-9713-9

Milady
5 Maxwell Drive
Clifton Park, NY 12065-2919
USA

Cengage Learning products are represented in Canada by
Nelson Education, Ltd.

For your lifelong learning solutions, visit **milady.cengage.com**

Visit our corporate website at **cengage.com**

Notice to the Reader
Publisher does not warrant or guarantee any of the products described herein or perform any independent analysis in connection with any of the product information contained herein. Publisher does not assume, and expressly disclaims, any obligation to obtain and include information other than that provided to it by the manufacturer. The reader is expressly warned to consider and adopt all safety precautions that might be indicated by the activities described herein and to avoid all potential hazards. By following the instructions contained herein, the reader willingly assumes all risks in connection with such instructions. The publisher makes no representations or warranties of any kind, including but not limited to, the warranties of fitness for particular purpose or merchantability, nor are any such representations implied with respect to the material set forth herein, and the publisher takes no responsibility with respect to such material. The publisher shall not be liable for any special, consequential, or exemplary damages resulting, in whole or part, from the readers' use of, or reliance upon, this material.

Printed in the United States of America
5 XX 14 13

Table of Contents

How To Use This Workbook

Milady's Standard Professional Barbering Student Workbook strengthens students' understanding of barbering by reinforcing material covered in the student textbook, *Milady's Standard Professional Barbering*, Fifth Edition.

This workbook contains short answer, short essay, sentence completion, matching, definition, and labeling activities. Word Reviews are supplied for each chapter and may be used as general study guides or to stimulate classroom discussions—or may be assigned by the instructor for use in creative essays and exercises.

Students should complete each workbook chapter as the textbook chapter is covered in class. Instructors should determine how the workbook material will be used as it applies to assignments or grades.

This workbook should be used in conjunction with *Milady's Standard Professional Barbering*, Fifth Edition.

Date: _____

Rating: _____

Text Pages 1–13

Chapter 1: Study Skills

Word Review

drafting	mind-mapping	planning
editing	mnemonics	repetition
learning styles	organization	revising

TOPIC 1: Introduction

1. How long has it been since you attended classes in an educational program?

   _____

2. What is one of the most important keys to your success as a student?

   _____

TOPIC 2: Study Skills

1. What are study skills?

   _____

   _____

2. Identify five information processing methods that can enhance and optimize studying efforts.

   _____

   _____

3. Match the following words with the correct definition or example.

   _____ note-taking   a) categorizing information into smaller segments

   _____ mind-mapping   b) saying or writing something several times

   _____ mnemonics   c) an illustration used to take notes or solve problems

   _____ organization   d) memory triggers using songs, acronyms, etc.

   _____ repetition   e) the writing down of key ideas or concepts

4. Outlining is a useful way to take notes because it helps to identify and organize key topics and associated details. Use the words in the "Think Tank" as many times as necessary to fill in the outline that follows.

Think Tank		
first main idea		detail
topic		subtopic
second main topic		third main topic

_____

I. _____

   A. _____

      1. _____

      2. _____

   B. _____

      1. _____

      2. _____

II. _____

   A. _____

   B. _____

III. _____

REPORT WRITING

1. The writing process has four distinct steps. They are _____, _____, _____, and _____.

2. Match the following words with the correct characteristic of the writing step.

   _____ planning   a) includes rewriting or reorganizing the material

   _____ drafting   b) involves proofreading and correcting the work

   _____ revising   c) includes formal outlining and sentence construction

   _____ editing   d) involves anything done prior to writing the first draft

TOPIC 3: Learning Styles

1. What are learning styles?

   _____

   _____

2. How does learning take place?

   _____

   _____

3. Perceptions of reality tend to be either more emotionally centered or more analytically based. Do you most often *feel* your way through new information or situations or *think* your way through new information or situations?

   _____

4. New information or experiences are usually processed through *watching* and *absorbing* or through *action* and *doing*. What is your preferred method of processing new information or experiences?

   _____

   _____

5. Four learning styles emerge when two different ways of _____ are combined with the two different ways of _____.

6. Review the following learning style types and then check the characteristics of each that best describe you. The learning type with the most checkmarks is your preferred learning style. Record it here.

_____

Interactive Learners I...	Reader/listener Learners I...
☐ Like to perceive information by experiencing it and then thinking about it.	☐ Like to perceive information by thinking about it and then thinking about it some more.
☐ Learn by listening and sharing ideas.	☐ Learn by reflecting and thinking on the topic.
☐ Value insightful thinking.	☐ Tend to form theories and concepts by integrating observations with what I know.
☐ View experiences from many perspectives.	☐ Like to know what the experts think.
☐ Love harmony.	☐ Am good at detail work.
☐ Am committed to tasks that I undertake and commit to.	☐ Like to work or learn in sequence.
☐ Like learning about people and cultures.	☐ Tend to ask the question, "What?"
☐ Enjoy studying in a group.	
☐ Tend to ask the question, "Why?"	

Systematic Learners I...	Intuitive Learners I...
☐ Like to perceive information by thinking about it, but I process information by doing things.	☐ Like to perceive information by experiencing it, and I process it actively.
☐ Tend to integrate theory and application.	☐ Tend to integrate experience and application.
☐ Learn best by testing theories and using common sense.	☐ Learn by trial and error.
☐ Like to problem-solve.	☐ Am adaptable and enjoy change.
☐ Value strategic thinking.	☐ Am a risk-taker.
☐ Am skills oriented.	☐ Take what is and add to it.
☐ Like to experiment with ideas and things.	☐ Am at ease with people.
☐ Like to get to the point.	☐ Believe in self-discovery.
☐ Tend to ask the question, "How?"	☐ Tend to ask the question, "What if...?"

TOPIC 4: Developing Effective Study Habits

1. To study effectively, you need to know _____, _____, _____, and _____ to study.

2. Identify your favorite time, place, and method to study.

   time: _____

   place: _____

   method: _____

3. The development of good study habits is a _____ skill that can be used throughout a lifetime to achieve personal and professional potential.

3

Chapter 2: The History of Barbering

Word Review

A. B. Moler
Associated Master Barbers
   and Beauticians of America
   (AMBBA)
Ambroise Pare
barba

barber-surgeons
journeymen barbers
master barbers
Meryma'at
National Association of Barber
   Boards of America

Ticinius Mena
tondere
tonsorial
tonsure

TOPIC 1: Introduction

1. The history of barbering and hairstyling is deeply rooted in the progress of mankind and barbering is one of the _____ professions in the world.

2. Barbering and hairstyling developed from _____ and _____ beginnings into a recognized profession.

TOPIC 2: Origin of the Barber

1. From what Latin word is the word *barber* derived and what does it mean?

   _____

2. What does the Latin-derived word *tonsorial* mean?

   _____

3. From what Latin word is the word *tonsure* derived and what does it mean?

   _____

4. What is a tonsure?

   _____

5. Match the following definitions or descriptions with the correct name or word.

_____ Egyptian coloring agent

_____ brought shaving and barbering services in Rome in 296 B.C.

_____ wore three braided sections and queues

_____ credited with cultivating beauty extravagantly

_____ barbers rose in prominence during this time

_____ decreed that his soldiers were to be clean-shaven

_____ hid his facial scars behind a beard

_____ what early hairstyles usually indicated

_____ the mark of dignity and manhood for Chinese men

_____ what the color of a Roman woman's hair indicated

_____ the circular tonsure decreed by the pope for clergymen

_____ abolished the practice of the tonsure in 1972

_____ wore gray wigs

_____ indicated political and religious affiliations in England

_____ believed hair to be the source of the brain's inspiration

_____ encouraged shaving by imposing a tax on beards

_____ the Egyptians created a statue in his honor

a) Emperor Hadrian

b) hairstyles

c) social status

d) class or rank

e) Ticinius Mena

f) Roman Catholic Church

g) henna

h) Pythagoras

i) Golden Age of Greece

j) Masai warriors

k) British barristers

l) Egyptians

m) Alexander the Great

n) queue

o) Meryma'at

p) Peter the Great

q) St. Peter

TOPIC 3: The Beard and Shaving

Because the practice of shaving pre-dates the written word, it is difficult to determine just when this form of hair removal began.

1. Artwork of the _____ period shows examples of clean-shaven men.

2. In early times, most groups considered the beard to be a sign of _____ , _____ , and _____ .

3. By 1000 B.C. _____ men were visiting the local barber for shaving services on a regular basis.

4. Provide two reasons why the common classes patronized the barbershops in addition to receiving shaving and haircutting services. _____

TOPIC 4: The Rise of the Barber-Surgeons

1. During the Middle Ages, barbers figured prominently in the development of _____ as a recognized branch of medical practice.

2. Barbers often assisted the clergy in the practice of _____ .

3. Barbers who practiced bloodletting, minor surgery, herbal remedies, and tooth-pulling were called _____ .

5

4. The _____ was ruled by a master and consisted of two classes of barbers: those who practiced _____ and those who specialized in _____.

5. The Company of Barber-Surgeons was granted a charter in 1540 by _____.

6. The barber-surgeon named _____ is considered the father of modern surgery.

7. _____ and _____ settlers brought barber-surgeons with them to America to look after the well-being of the colonists.

8. The symbol of the barber-surgeons is the _____.

9. The symbol of the barber pole evolved from the technical procedure of _____.

10. When the Barber Surgeon's Company in England was formed, barbers were required to use _____ and white poles, whereas surgeons used _____ and white poles.

11. The red, white, and blue barber poles displayed in the United States may have originated

_____.

TOPIC 5: Modern Barbers and Barbering

By the nineteenth century, barbering was completely separated from religion and medicine and began to emerge as an independent profession.

1. Match the following definitions or descriptions with the correct name or word.

_____ employee groups

_____ employer groups

_____ year and location of the formation of the journeymen barbers' union

_____ year and location associated with the opening of America's first barber school

_____ year the first Moler manual of barbering was first published

_____ the first state to pass barber licensing laws

_____ the year and location the Associated Master Barbers of America was formed

_____ the group the AMBBA represented

_____ standardized and upgraded barber training

_____ standardized the operation of barber schools

_____ National Association of State Board of Barber Examiners

_____ adopted a barber code of ethics

_____ the only state that does not regulate barbering

a) National Educational Council

b) National Association of Barber Schools

c) AMBBA

d) journeymen barbers

e) Alabama

f) 1893, Chicago, Illinois

g) master barbers

h) organized in St. Paul, Minnesota

i) 1924, Chicago, Illinois

j) 1893

k) 1887, New York

l) shop and salon owners

m) Minnesota

2. Some of the changes that have improved the practice of barbering within the last century are:

a) _____

_____

b) _____

_____

c) _____

_____

d) _____

_____

e) _____

_____

f) _____

_____

Date: _____

Rating: _____

Text Pages 32–52

Chapter 3: Professional Image

Word Review

attitude	goal setting	rapport
beliefs	life skills	receptivity
compartmentalization	motivation	self-management
diplomacy	personal hygiene	values
ergonomics	personality	
ethics	professional image	

TOPIC 1: Introduction

1. All of us are unique and complex individuals; our _____ and _____ make each of us who we are.

2. Factors that have the ability to influence and impact our professional image originate from _____.

TOPIC 2: Professional Image

1. The impression that you project as a person engaged in the profession of barbering is known as your _____.

2. Your professional image consists of the outward appearance, attitude, and conduct that you exhibit in the _____.

3. Tools and guidelines that prepare you for living as a mature adult are called _____.

4. Life skills are developed through _____ and _____.

5. Review the following list of life skills. Use a checkmark (✓) to indicate the life skills you feel you have mastered and an "x" next to the ones you feel you need to improve or enhance.

   ☐ showing genuine concern and caring for other people

   ☐ adapting to different situations

   ☐ developing and achieving goals

   ☐ showing persistence and a "can do" attitude

   ☐ following through with and completing jobs, tasks, and commitments

   ☐ developing and using common sense

   ☐ establishing positive and healthy relationships

   ☐ approaching everything with a strong sense of responsibility and a positive attitude

   ☐ feeling good about yourself

   ☐ being cooperative

8

☐ being organized

☐ maintaining a sense of humor

☐ being patient with yourself and others

☐ being honest and trustworthy

☐ striving for excellence

6. Attitudes originate from the two personal characteristics of _____ and _____.

7. _____ are the deepest feelings and thoughts we have about ourselves and about life.

8. _____ are specific attitudes that occur as a result of our values and have a strong influence on how we act or behave in situations.

9. When something comes true simply because you think it will come true, it is called a _____.

10. A positive self-fulfilling prophecy to inspire change, to take action, or to make a commitment to goals can be achieved by substituting _____ for _____.

TOPIC 3: Personality

Your personality plays an important role in both your personal and professional life.

1. Personality can be defined as the _____ of inner feelings, thoughts, attitudes, and values.

2. Personality is expressed through voice, _____, choice of words, _____, _____, gestures, _____, posture, clothing, _____, and environment.

3. Your personality _____ who you are and distinguishes you from others.

4. Your personality demonstrates your particular style of _____.

TOPIC 4: Attitude

Attitudes stem from innate values and beliefs, but may change with new insights.

1. The extent to which others or situations are allowed to change one's attitude depends on the _____.

2. A person's attitude is one of the most obvious and apparent aspects of their _____.

3. Match the following descriptions with the correct word(s).

_____ controlled, even-tempered emotions   a) courtesy

_____ being responsive to other's ideas and feelings   b) sensitivity

_____ reflects thoughtfulness of others   c) receptivity

_____ shows understanding, empathy, and acceptance   d) diplomacy

_____ the art of being tactful   e) emotional stability

9

TOPIC 5: Personal and Professional Health

In accordance with the general concept of the profession of helping others to look their best, barbers should strive to reflect their own best image.

1. The branch of applied science concerned with healthful living is called _____.

2. _____ is the daily maintenance of cleanliness and healthfulness through certain sanitary practices.

3. A _____ barber is one of the best advertisements for the barbershop.

4. Body tissues and organs are rebuilt and renewed during the _____ process.

5. The nutrients in food supply the body with _____ and ensure that the body functions properly.

6. _____ helps to develop the muscles and keep the body fit.

7. Exercise improves organ _____ and blood _____.

8. The inability to cope with a real or imagined threat that results in a series of mental and physical responses or adaptations is known as _____.

9. Stress management routines provide time to calm the body and its _____.

10. The body and mind operate as a unit; therefore, thoughts may either _____ or _____ the way the body functions.

11. _____ lessens fatigue and the possibility of other physical problems.

12. Repetitive motions used in barbering can create physical stress in the hands, wrists, arms, shoulders, and lower back areas. What are some methods that can be used to help prevent or reduce the occurrence of these possible conditions?

   a) _____

   b) _____

   c) _____

   d) _____

   e) _____

   f) _____

   g) _____

   h) _____

13. What are some guidelines for a correct sitting posture?

   a) _____

   b) _____

   c) _____

d) _____

e) _____

f) _____
   _____

14. _____ is the study of human characteristics for the specific work environment.

15. Complete the following suggestions that will help you fit your work to your body more effectively.

   a) Do not grip or squeeze _____ and _____ too tightly.

   b) Do not bend the _____ up or down constantly when cutting hair or using a blow-dryer.

   c) Try to position your arms at less than a _____-degree angle when holding your arms away from your body while working.

   d) Avoid _____ or _____ your body.

   e) Wear appropriate and supportive _____ or footwear.

   f) Adjust the _____ of the chair so the client's head is at a comfortable working level.

   g) Tilt the _____ as necessary for better access during hair services.

   h) Keep your wrists in a straight or _____ position as much as possible.

   i) Keep tools and implements _____ and well lubricated.

TOPIC 6: Human Relations

Effective human relations skills help you to build rapport with clients and coworkers.

1. _____ is the psychology of getting along well with others.

2. A close and empathetic relationship that establishes agreement and harmony between individuals is known as _____.

3. The following guidelines for good human relations will help you to gain confidence, deal courteously with others, and become a successful professional. Use a checkmark (✓) to indicate the human relations skills you feel you have mastered and an "x" next to the skills you feel you need to improve or enhance.

   ☐ Always greet a client or coworker by name, using a pleasant tone of voice.

   ☐ Be alert to clients' and coworkers' moods.

   ☐ Be a good listener.

   ☐ Never gossip or tell off-color stories.

   ☐ Choose topics of conversation carefully.

   ☐ Always maintain an ethical standard of confidentiality.

   ☐ Make a good impression by looking the part of a successful barber.

   ☐ Speak and act in a professional manner at all times.

- ☐ Cultivate self-confidence and project a pleasing personality.
- ☐ Show interest in the client's personal preferences and give undivided attention.
- ☐ Use tact and diplomacy when dealing with problems.
- ☐ Deal with all disputes and differences in private.
- ☐ Take care of all problems promptly and to the client's satisfaction.
- ☐ Be capable and efficient.
- ☐ Be punctual.
- ☐ Talk less, listen more.
- ☐ Practice emotional control.
- ☐ Have a positive approach.
- ☐ Practice good manners.
- ☐ Avoid annoying mannerisms (gum chewing, nervous habits, etc.).

TOPIC 7: Effective Communication Skills

Effective communication is one of the barber's most important human relations skills.

1. Communication includes listening skills, voice, speech, and _____ ability.

2. Communication is the act of transmitting information in the form of symbols, gestures, or behaviors to express an idea or concept so that it is clearly understood. What are three steps you can take to ascertain a client's service expectations?

   a) _____

   b) _____

   c) _____

3. There are certain topics that are suitable for conversation in the barbershop. Review the following list and check the topics you think are appropriate.

   - ☐ client's grooming needs
   - ☐ religion
   - ☐ sports
   - ☐ civic affairs
   - ☐ books or music
   - ☐ client's sex problems
   - ☐ your own problems
   - ☐ vacation plans
   - ☐ styling products
   - ☐ shop marketing promotions

4. There are certain behaviors by the barber that a client may find annoying. Review the following list and check the actions that you think would be annoying to a client.

☐ talking continuously

☐ listening intently

☐ gossiping

☐ talking to the barber next to you

☐ taking phone calls while working on the client

☐ being prompt

☐ swearing

☐ using poor English and grammar

TOPIC 8: Professional Ethics

Ethics are the principles and standards of good character, proper conduct, and moral judgment.

1. In barbering, ethics is a _____, which is expressed through personality, human relation skills, and professional image.

2. A _____ relates specifically to the characteristics of a particular profession.

3. Can you tell the difference between good and poor ethical practices on the job? Rate each of the following statements with a "G" or "P" as examples of either good or poor ethical behavior.

_____ a) having a sincere belief in barbering

_____ b) showing favoritism to some clients

_____ c) maintaining a good reputation

_____ d) giving the best possible service

_____ e) selling a client a product he does not need

_____ f) disobeying barbering laws

_____ g) keeping your word

_____ h) being loyal to your employer

_____ i) making extravagant claims

_____ j) practicing sanitation procedures

TOPIC 9: The Psychology of Success

Basic principles that form the foundation of personal and professional success include building self-esteem, learning to visualize, building on your strengths, and being kind to yourself.

1. List additional principles that help to attain personal and professional success.

a) _____

b) _____

c) _____

d) _____

e) _____

f) _____

g) _____

You are in charge of managing your own life and learning.

2. _____ originates from a desire for change and serves as the ignition for success.

3. A well-thought-out process for achieving goals in the long term is called _____.

4. _____ blocks the creative mind from exploring ideas and discovering solutions to challenges.

5. Turning dreams into reality is what _____ is all about.

6. Goals to be attained in a year or less are considered _____ goals.

7. Goal setting is a _____ that requires planning.

8. An "inner organizer" refers to _____.

9. _____ tasks in order of most to least important.

10. Learn _____ techniques to save time when seeking solutions.

14

Chapter 4: Microbiology

Word Review

acquired immunity
acquired immunodeficiency
    syndrome (AIDS)
active (vegetative) stage
aseptic
bacilli
bacteria
bloodborne pathogens
cocci
contagious (communicable)
diplococci
flagella
fungi
general infection

hepatitis
human disease carrier
human immunodeficiency
    virus (HIV)
immunity
inactive stage
infection
local infection
mitosis
methicillin-resistant
    Staphylococcus aureus
    (MRSA)
natural immunity
nonpathogenic

objective symptoms
parasites
pathogenic
pediculosis
pus
scabies
sepsis
spirilla
spore-forming bacteria
staphylococci
streptococci
subjective symptoms
virus

TOPIC 1: Introduction

Each year the barbering industry services hundreds of thousands of clients. That means barbers and their clients are exposed to billions of microorganisms in the form of bacteria, viruses, or parasites that may result in illness or infection.

1. It is the barber's responsibility to ensure that clients receive services in a _____ and _____ environment.

2. Contagious diseases, skin infections, and blood poisoning can be caused by the transmission of infectious material from one individual to another or through the use of unsanitary _____ and _____.

TOPIC 2: Microbiology

1. Microbiology is the branch of science that studies living organisms, known as _____ or _____, too small to be seen with the naked eye.

2. Microorganisms are generally classified as _____, _____, _____, _____, or _____.

3. Microorganisms capable of causing infectious diseases in plants or animals are called _____.

TOPIC 3: Bacteriology

1. Bacteriology is the science that deals with the study of _____ called bacteria.

2. Bacteria are also known as _____ or _____.

3. Bacteria are minute, _____ microorganisms that exist almost everywhere.

4. Bacteria can only be seen with the aid of a _____.

The many different kinds of bacteria are classified into two general types: nonpathogenic and pathogenic bacteria.

5. _____ bacteria are beneficial or harmless and perform many useful functions such as decomposing refuse and improving the fertility of the soil.

6. _____ bacteria are harmful and cause disease by invading plant or human tissues.

7. Pathogenic bacteria are classified as _____ , _____ , or _____ .

8. Match the following definitions or words to the correct bacteria type.

_____ short, rod-shaped microorganisms   a) bacilli

_____ round-shaped microorganisms   b) streptococci

_____ corkscrew-shaped microorganisms   c) cocci

_____ microorganisms that grow in bunches or clusters   d) diplococci

_____ microorganisms that grow in chains   e) spirilla

_____ microorganisms that grow in pairs   f) staphylococci

9. Match the following diseases to the bacteria that produce them. Bacteria choices may be used more than once.

_____ abscesses and pustules   a) cocci

_____ strep throat   b) bacilli

_____ pneumonia   c) spirilla

_____ syphilis   d) staphylococci

_____ blood poisoning   e) streptococci

_____ diphtheria   f) diplococci

_____ boils

_____ gonorrhea

_____ tonsillitis

_____ tetanus

_____ Lyme disease

_____ MRSA (methicillin-resistant *Staphylococcus aureus*)

10. _____ rarely show active motility. They are transmitted in the air, in dust, or within the substances in which they settle.

11. Bacilli and spirilla are both motile and use hair-like projections, known as _____ or cilia, to move about.

12. Bacteria have two distinct phases in their life cycle: the active or _____ stage and the _____ stage.

13. During the _____ or _____ stage, bacteria grow and reproduce.

14. The division of cells during growth and reproduction is called _____.

15. The cells that are formed when cells divide are called _____.

16. During the _____ stage, bacteria do not _____ or reproduce. They may lie dormant until conditions are favorable for reproduction or _____ off.

17. Some bacteria, such as the anthrax and tetanus bacilli, may survive the inactive stage by forming spherical or round _____ with tough outer coverings. In this stage, spores are not harmed by most _____, heat, or cold.

TOPIC 4: Bacterial Infections

1. An _____ occurs if the body is unable to cope with bacteria and their harmful toxins.

2. The presence of _____ is a sign of infection.

3. Match the following definitions with the correct word or words. Word choices may be used more than once.

_____ indicated by a lesion containing pus

_____ the bloodstream carries bacteria through the body

_____ pimples and boils

_____ can cause an epidemic

_____ usually appears in a particular area of the body

_____ caused by toxins carried through the body

_____ disease spreads from one person to another

_____ disease that attacks a large group simultaneously

a) communicable

b) local infection

c) general infection

d) epidemic

4. List some of the more contagious diseases or disorders that will prevent a barber from servicing clients.

a) _____

b) _____

c) _____

d) _____

e) _____

f) _____

TOPIC 5: Bloodborne Pathogens

1. Disease-producing bacteria or viruses that are carried through the body in blood or body fluids are called _____.

2. Blood-to-blood contact might occur if blood from a one person's cut is transmitted through a contaminated _____ to someone else's cut or wound.

3. Body fluids, such as pus, can be picked up from a _____ or open sore when using razors or clippers.

4. Pathogenic bacteria or viruses may enter the body through:

   a) _____

   b) _____

   c) _____

   d) _____

   e) _____

5. The body fights infection by means of its defensive forces. These include (a) _____ skin, (b) body secretions, (c) _____ blood cells, and (d) antitoxins.

6. Infections created by pathogenic bacteria or viruses can be controlled through _____ and public sanitation.

TOPIC 6: Terminology

1. Match the following word or words to the most correct definition. Word choices may be used more than once.

   _____ freedom from disease germs

   _____ signs of disease

   _____ poisoning due to pathogenic bacteria

   _____ symptoms that are seen

   _____ symptoms that are felt

   _____ organisms that live on another living organism

   _____ molds and mildews

   _____ itch mite

   _____ yeasts

   _____ lice

   _____ ringworm

   _____ the body's resistance to bacteria

   _____ partially inherited/developed immunity

   _____ immunity developed after overcoming a disease

   _____ immunity developed after inoculation

   _____ immunity developed through hygienic living

   _____ a person immune to a disease, but who can infect others

   a) plant parasite
   b) subjective
   c) asepsis
   d) animal parasite
   e) sepsis
   f) objective
   g) symptoms
   h) parasites
   i) acquired immunity
   j) human disease carrier
   k) immunity
   l) natural immunity

18

TOPIC 7: Viruses

1. Viruses are capable of infecting almost all plants, animals, and _____.

2. Viruses live only by penetrating cells and becoming a part of them and are generally resistant to _____.

3. _____ and _____ are examples of bloodborne pathogens.

TOPIC 8: Hepatitis

Hepatitis is a bloodborne virus, present in all body fluids, that causes disease marked by inflammation of the liver.

1. While there are several types of hepatitis virus, three types found in the United States are the _____, _____, and _____ viruses.

2. Review the following list and check those symptoms that apply to one or more hepatitis conditions.

   - ☐ flu-like symptoms
   - ☐ fatigue
   - ☐ nausea
   - ☐ fever
   - ☐ abdominal pain
   - ☐ loss of appetite

3. Review the following list and check those methods of transmission that apply to one or more hepatitis conditions.

   - ☐ poor sanitation
   - ☐ poor personal hygiene
   - ☐ common bathroom use
   - ☐ contaminated foods and liquids
   - ☐ sexual contact
   - ☐ blood products and saliva
   - ☐ parenteral exposure to blood or blood products
   - ☐ blood transfusions with contaminated blood
   - ☐ illegal drug injections

4. There are no vaccines available for the hepatitis _____, _____, and _____ viruses.

TOPIC 9: HIV/AIDS

The human immunodeficiency virus is the virus that causes acquired immunodeficiency syndrome (AIDS). AIDS is the onset of life-threatening illnesses that compromise the immune system as a result of HIV infection and disease.

1. _____ is passed from person to person through body fluids such as blood, breast milk, semen, and vaginal secretions.

2. A person can be infected with HIV for up to _____ without having symptoms.

3. HIV can enter the bloodstream through cuts and sores and may be transmitted in the barbershop through _____ implements.

4. HIV may lie dormant in an infected person's system for _____ years or more. It can also mature into a fatal disease in _____ to _____ years.

5. The fact that the HIV uses the reproductive processes of the host cell to duplicate itself means that it is a _____.

6. Once the HIV has entered the bloodstream and the immune response begins, antibodies will normally be produced within a range of _____ to _____.

7. HIV goes through several stages before it becomes full-blown AIDS. Review the following list of symptoms then, match the conditions to the first stage in which the symptoms are presented.

   _____ chronic fatigue   a) Stage 1—HIV infection

   _____ skin/other cancers   b) Stage 2—AIDS-related complex (ARC)

   _____ swollen lymph glands   c) Stage 3—AIDS

   _____ no physical indications

   _____ hair loss

   _____ weight loss without dieting

   _____ antibodies may be present

   _____ nerve damage

   _____ night sweats

   _____ enlarged liver/spleen

   _____ pneumonia

8. To date, there is no _____ to prevent HIV infection, nor is there a _____ for AIDS.

9. An _____ test should be performed on persons who think they may be at risk for HIV.

10. Bacteria may be destroyed through the use of _____, _____, and _____.

Chapter 5: Infection Control and Safe Work Practices

Word Review

antiseptics
blood-spill disinfection
decontamination
disinfectants
disinfection
dry (cabinet) sanitizer
efficacy
Environmental Protection
    Agency (EPA)
EPA-registered disinfectants
exposure incident

Food and Drug Administration
    (FDA)
Hazard Communication Rule
hospital-grade tuberculocidal
    disinfectant
hospital level disinfectant
Material Safety Data Sheet(s)
Occupational Safety and Health
    Administration (OSHA)
Occupational Safety and
    Health Act

public sanitation
Right-to-Know Law
safe work practices
sanitation
solute
solution
solvent
standard precautions
sterilization
ultraviolet-ray sanitizer
wet sanitizer

TOPIC 1: Introduction

State barber boards and health departments require that sanitary measures be applied while serving the public.

1. Infection control measures help to minimize the spread of contagious diseases, skin infections, and _____ that can be caused by the transmission of infectious material from one individual to another or through the use of _____ combs, clippers, razors, shears, or other barbering tools and implements.

2. Professional barbers employ _____ methods to help safeguard their health and the health of their clients.

3. Safe work practices relate to an awareness of the potential hazards that can exist in the barbershop and strategies that help _____ associated risks.

4. Barbers are responsible for employing safe work practices that help prevent accidents and injury from occurring in the _____.

TOPIC 2: Regulation

1. _____ agencies set guidelines for the protection of human health and the environment, and safe work practices for most occupational and manufacturing sectors.

2. State and local agencies _____ and _____ licensing, minimum standards, workplace conduct, and other oversight responsibilities to ensure public health and safety.

3. The _____ and each individual state must approve disinfectants used in the workplace.

4. The _____ is responsible for enforcing rules and regulations associated with food, drug, and cosmetic products purchased and used by the _____.

5. Hair tonics, shampoos, conditioners, permanent wave solutions, hair color tints, chemical processors, hairsprays, and gels used in the barbershop are called _____ preparations.

6. _____ products are those that are sold only to licensed barbers or other industry professionals.

7. _____'s primary purpose is to assure, regulate, and enforce safe and healthful working conditions in the workplace.

8. Three federal agencies that help regulate infection control and safe work practices in the barbershop are the _____, _____, and _____.

9. Two important results of the Hazard Communication Rule are _____ and required _____.

10. The purpose of an MSDS is to provide vital information about product _____, associated _____, combustion levels, and storage requirements.

11. Barbershops and schools are required by law to maintain an _____ for every product used on the premises.

12. The listing of ingredients with appropriate hazard warnings on the packaging of a product is called _____.

13. The intent of the _____ is to inform employees of toxic substances in the workplace and to advise them of their rights.

14. It is the responsibility of the _____ to inform workers of toxic substances in the workplace.

TOPIC 3: Decontamination

1. The removal of pathogens and other substances from tools or surfaces is called _____.

2. Decontamination involves the use of _____ or _____ processes to remove, inactivate, or destroy pathogens to make an object safe for handling, use, or disposal.

3. The term _____ means to thoroughly clean an item or surface with soap or detergents and water, and refers to the _____ step in the disinfection process.

4. *Disinfect* means to thoroughly _____ a surface or item followed by the application of a chemical _____.

5. The three main levels of decontamination are _____, _____, and _____.

6. State barber boards and health departments require _____ and _____ procedures to be performed in the barbershop environment.

7. _____ is the application of measures to promote public health and prevent the spread of infectious diseases.

22

8. Room temperature in the barbershop should be about _____ degrees Fahrenheit.

9. Many municipal governments require _____ in establishments that serve the general public.

10. Match the following definitions with the most correct word or words. Choices may be used more than once.

_____ significantly reduces pathogens on a surface	a) sterilization
_____ destroys all living organisms on a surface	b) disinfection
_____ wastewater management	c) sanitation, sanitizing, or cleansing
_____ destroys most bacteria and some viruses	d) public sanitation
_____ second only to sterilization	
_____ lowest level of decontamination	
_____ pollution control	
_____ process of cleaning and disinfecting a tool/surface	
_____ requires steaming, boiling, or baking	
_____ garbage removal	
_____ washing with soap and water	
_____ requires the use of chemical disinfectants	
_____ highest level of decontamination	

11. Moist heat (boiling water), steaming (autoclave), dry heat, and ultraviolet rays are examples of _____ agents.

12. An ultraviolet-ray electric sanitizer will keep _____ tools and implements _____ until they are removed for use.

13. _____ agents are the most effective sanitizing and disinfecting methods used in barbershops to destroy or check the spread of pathogenic bacteria.

14. _____ may kill, retard, or prevent the growth of bacteria and can generally be used safely on the skin.

15. Chemical agents that destroy most bacteria and some viruses are _____; they should not be used on the _____, _____, or _____.

16. The four levels of disinfection efficacy among EPA-registered disinfectants are _____, _____, _____, and _____.

17. To perform the optimum level of disinfection, disinfectants must be effective against _____, _____, _____, _____, _____, _____, and _____. The ability to combat these organisms places this type of disinfectant into the _____ disinfectant group.

18. Match the following definitions with the most correct word or words. Word choices may be used more than once.

_____ common household bleach

_____ releases formaldehyde gas

_____ quaternary ammonium compounds

_____ may eliminate or minimize rust formation

_____ product recommending a 10 percent solution and a 10-minute immersion time

_____ uses a 1:1000 solution

_____ may soften or discolor rubber and plastic

_____ is an organic compound

_____ used on clippers and trimmers

_____ used for general cleaning purposes

_____ its use may be prohibited

_____ should contain a rust inhibitor

a) quats

b) phenols

c) commercial cleaners

d) prepared commercial products

e) sodium hypochlorite

f) alcohol

g) formalin

h) petroleum distillates

19. A _____ is the product resulting from dissolving a solute in a solvent. The _____ is the substance that is dissolved and the _____ is the liquid in which a solute is dissolved.

20. A 10 percent bleach solution means that 10 percent of the solution is _____ and 90 percent is _____ .

21. Mixing chemicals stronger than recommended by the manufacturer may counteract the _____ of the product.

22. Dry cabinet sanitizers require an active _____ to be effective as disinfecting units and are rarely used in today's barbershops.

23. A _____ is a covered receptacle large enough to hold a disinfectant solution into which objects can be completely immersed.

24. _____ sanitizers are cabinets with ultraviolet bulbs used to store sanitized tools and implements.

TOPIC 4: Disinfection Procedures

1. Review and order the following list of procedures from 1 to 9 in the correct procedural order.

_____ Wash item(s) thoroughly with hot water and soap.

_____ Store item(s) in a dry cabinet sanitizer, ultraviolet sanitizer, or covered container until needed.

_____ Remove item(s) from the disinfectant and rinse thoroughly.

_____ Read manufacturer's directions for disinfectant solution and mix accordingly.

_____ Dry item(s) with a clean towel.

_____ Disinfect for the recommended time.

_____ Rinse item(s) thoroughly and pat dry.

_____ Place item(s) in wet sanitizer containing disinfectant solution; immerse completely.

_____ Remove hair from combs, brushes, etc.

2. Procedures for implement immersion into a chemical solution must conform to the _____, _____, and/or _____ regulations in your state.

3. The cleaning of tools and implements prior to disinfectant immersion helps to avoid _____ of the solution.

4. Products containing a petroleum distillate, such as liquid blade washes, are the usual choice for the decontamination of clippers and trimmers.

5. Review and order the following list of procedures from 1 to 7 in the correct procedural order.

_____ Arrange all supplies, products, and tools on a clean, sanitized surface.

_____ Pour blade wash into a glass, plastic, or disposable container wide enough to accommodate the width of the clipper blades to a depth of approximately ½ inch.

_____ Spray with a blade lubricant and/or spray clipper disinfectant; grease/oil clipper parts.

_____ Submerge only the cutting teeth of the clipper blades into the blade wash and turn the unit on. Run until no hair particles are seen being dislodged from the blades.

_____ Store in a clean, closed container until needed for use.

_____ Remove the clippers and wipe blades with a clean, dry towel.

_____ Remove hair particles from clipper blades with a stiff brush.

6. Disinfecting station work surfaces includes counter-tops, barber chairs, armrests, _____, _____, and other surfaces.

7. _____ is one the most important and easiest ways to prevent the spread of germs from one person to another.

TOPIC 5: Standard (Universal) Precautions

Standard precautions are a set of guidelines and controls published by the Centers for Disease Control that require employers and employees to assume that all human blood and body fluids are infectious for HIV, HBV, and other bloodborne pathogens.

1. Standard precautions include:

   a) _____ washing

   b) Proper disinfection and _____ of tools

   c) Protective equipment such as _____ and goggles

d) Injury _____

e) Proper handling and disposal of sharp implements or _____ dressings.

2. An _____, formerly known as a blood spill, is the contact with _____ skin, _____, body fluid, or other potentially infectious materials that may occur during the performance of an individual's work duties.

3. Exposure incidents require _____ decontamination procedures be followed.

4. Fill in the blanks to complete the procedural steps that should be used when a client sustains a cut or nick in the performance of barbering services.

a) Stop the service _____ and _____ the client.

b) Wash your hands and apply _____.

c) _____ the injured area.

d) Apply antiseptic or styptic powder using a _____.

e) _____ with an appropriate dressing.

f) Discard all disposable contaminated objects by _____ and deposit sharp disposables in a _____.

g) _____ tools and workstation.

h) Remove gloves carefully and _____.

i) Wash your hands _____ returning to the service.

j) Reminder: Disinfect tools and implements that have come into contact with blood or body fluids in an EPA-registered _____.

5. Fill in the blanks to complete the procedural steps that should be used when the barber sustains a cut or minor injury.

a) Stop the service and _____ for possible transmission of blood.

b) Wash your _____.

c) Apply antiseptic or styptic using a cotton swab. Do not contaminate the _____.

d) Cover the injury with an appropriate dressing and/or _____ as necessary.

e) Discard all disposable contaminated objects by double-bagging. Use the appropriate _____ sticker on a container for contaminated waste. Deposit sharp disposables in a sharps box.

f) Disinfect _____ and workstation.

6. Barbers should wash their hands with a liquid _____ soap and warm water.

TOPIC 6: Safe Work Practices

Safe work practices include the maintenance of sanitation standards and the application of safety precautions in the workplace environment.

1. List the safety precaution areas or topics that are relevant to the barbershop environment.

    a) _____

    b) _____

    c) _____

    d) _____

    e) _____

    f) _____

    g) _____

    h) _____

    i) _____

    j) _____

    k) _____

2. A barber's professional _____ far exceed the requirement to perform a good haircut.

27

Chapter 6: Implements, Tools, and Equipment

Word Review

blades
changeable-blade straight razor
clippers
comedone extractor
conventional straight razor
guards
high-frequency machine

hone
palming the comb
palming the shears
rotary motor clipper
Russian strop
set of the shears
shell strop

strop
taper comb
thermal styling tools
thinning shears
trimmers

TOPIC 1: Introduction

Barbers should always use high-quality implements, tools, and equipment. When taken care of properly, well-tempered metal implements and electric tools will provide years of dependable service.

1. An example of an implement is _____.

2. An example of a tool is _____.

3. An example of equipment is _____.

TOPIC 2: Combs and Brushes

1. The principal tools used by barbers are combs, brushes, _____,
_____, _____, and _____.

2. Most barbers prefer combs made of _____.

3. The _____ of the comb should have rounded ends to avoid scratching a client's scalp.

4. The correct comb choice depends on the type of _____ to be
_____ and the individual _____ of the barber.

5. Match the following applications or purposes to the correct comb style.

_____ used for a gradual blending; has a narrow end   a) tail comb

_____ used with clippers for flat top styles   b) wide-toothed handle comb

_____ used for general haircutting and styling   c) taper comb

_____ used for sectioning and parting   d) pick or Afro comb

_____ used on tight curl patterns   e) wide-toothed comb

_____ may be used for detangling   f) all-purpose comb

6. Barbers can simplify their work when cutting hair by using _____ combs on dark hair and _____ combs on light hair.

28

7. Styling brushes are used to smooth, wave, or add fullness to hair or to _____ the scalp.

8. The type of brush used will depend on the _____ to be achieved and the barber's personal preference.

9. _____ bristle brushes clean hair by trapping particles and disperse _____ throughout the hair strands.

10. Brushes are cleaned and disinfected in the same manner as _____ .

TOPIC 3: Shears

1. The two types of shears generally used by barbers are the _____ style, which has a brace for the little finger, and the _____ type, which does not have a finger brace.

2. Label the parts of the shears in the following illustration.

3. Shears are measured in inches and _____ inches.

4. Most barbers prefer _____ inch shears.

5. The grind of the shear refers to the inside construction of the _____ and the way it is cut in preparation for sharpening and polishing. Two types of blade grinds are the _____ and _____ .

6. Blade _____ may be beveled, convex, or hybrid in design.

7. The _____ of the shears refers to the angle and alignment of the blades.

8. Thinning shears are also known as _____ , _____ , or texturizing shears and are used to reduce hair thickness or to create special texturizing effects.

9. When shears are closed and resting in the palm while combing through the hair, this is called _____ .

10. The tension of the shears depends on how tight or loose the tension _____ is set.

TOPIC 4: Clippers & Trimmers

Clippers and trimmers are two of the most important tools used in barbering.

1. Trimmers are also known as _____ or _____ and are essential for finish and detail work.

2. Some factors that should be considered when purchasing a clipper are _____, _____, _____, _____, and _____.

3. Some clippers have a detachable blade system, while others have an _____ blade.

4. Label the parts of the clipper in the following illustration.

5. The rotary motor clipper is also known as the _____ motor clipper.

6. The universal motor clipper has _____ clipper blades.

7. _____ motor clippers are twice as powerful as magnetic motor clippers.

8. The blades are pulled both ways in a _____ motor clipper.

9. Pivot motor clippers have an _____ blade controlled by a _____.

10. Vibratory or _____ clippers operate by means of an alternating spring and magnet mechanism.

11. Magnetic motor clippers run faster than rotary motor clippers and usually have _____ clipper blades.

12. An outliner may use a _____ or _____ motor.

13. Trimmers have a very fine cutting head for _____, _____, and _____ work.

14. _____ clippers are designed to rest in a recharging unit.

15. Clipper _____ are usually made of high-quality carbon steel and are available in a variety of styles and sizes.

16. Clipper _____ are most often made of plastic or hard rubber.

17. Never adjust clipper or trimmer blades _____ to each other.

TOPIC 5: Straight Razors

As the sharpest and closest cutting tool, razors are used for facial shaves, neck shaves, finish work around the sideburn and behind-the-ear areas, and haircutting. The razor of choice for professional barbering is the straight razor.

1. There are two types of straight razors: the _____-blade straight razor and the _____ straight razor.

2. The conventional straight razor requires _____ and _____ to maintain its cutting edge.

3. Selecting the right kind of razor is a matter of personal choice, but avoid judging a razor simply on _____ or _____ .

4. Label the parts of the razor in the following illustration.

5. The _____-blade straight razor eliminates honing and stropping, saves time, is usually lighter, and helps to maintain sanitation standards.

6. Always follow the _____ directions for inserting a new blade or removing an old blade from a changeable-blade razor.

7. The _____ straight razor is made of a hardened steel blade attached to a handle by means of a pivot.

8. To determine the quality of a razor, the following factors must be considered: razor

_____ , _____ , _____ , _____ ,

_____ , and _____ .

9. Match the following definitions with the most correct words. Word choices may be used more
   than once.

   _____ involves a special heat treatment

   _____ shape of the blade after grinding

   _____ polish of the razor surface

   _____ length and width of the blade

   _____ weight and length of blade relative to handle

   _____ blade and handle are equal

   _____ degree of hardness

   _____ concave and wedge

   _____ ⅝" and ⁹⁄₁₆"

   _____ crocus (polished steel)

   _____ shape and design

   a) razor grind

   b) razor temper

   c) razor balance

   d) razor finish

   e) razor size

   f) razor style

10. When closing the razor, be careful that the cutting edge does not strike the

    _____ .

TOPIC 6: Hones and Strops

1. Two vital accessories used with conventional straight razors are the _____ and
   the _____ .

2. A _____ is an abrasive material that has the ability to cut steel.
   A _____ is made of leather and canvas.

3. The _____ hone is a slow-cutting hone.

4. _____ hones consist of both a water hone and a synthetic hone.

5. The Swaty hone and the carborundum hone are types of _____ hones.

6. Hones are designed to _____ the edge of a razor into a sharp cutting edge; strops
   are used to smooth and _____ the razor.

7. Strops are categorized as French or German, canvas, cowhide, _____ , or imitation
   leather.

8. Match the following definitions with the correct word. Word choices may be used more than once.

_____ combined strop with leather and finishing strop   a) imitation leather strop

_____ originally imported from Russia   b) Russian shell strop

_____ made from the rump area of a horse   c) cowhide strop

_____ not satisfactory for barbershop use   d) canvas strop

_____ requires little breaking in   e) French or German strop

_____ made of linen or silk

9. _____ cleans the leather strop, preserves its finish, and improves its draw and sharpening qualities.

10. When honing a razor, the strokes must be even in _____, _____, and _____ on both sides of the blade.

11. The hone should be kept _____ while in use.

12. A honed razor should never be used for shaving without first being _____.

13. The direction of the razor used in stropping is the _____ of the direction used in honing.

14. A properly stropped razor will have a sharp drawing sensation when passed over a moistened thumb; a _____ edge does not produce a drawing sensation.

TOPIC 7: Additional Barbering Implements, Tools, and Equipment

1. Match the following definitions with the correct implement, tool, or equipment.

_____ appliance used in shaving services   a) thermal styling irons and combs

_____ contain natural or artificial bristles   b) comedone extractor

_____ used to remove hair clippings   c) blow-dryer

_____ used to dry and style hair   d) electric latherizer

_____ uses heat to curl or straighten hair   e) hot towel cabinet

_____ introduces water-soluble products into skin   f) electric vibrator or massager

_____ used with glass electrodes   g) electric hair vacuum

_____ warms towels for barbering services   h) high-frequency machine

_____ used to press out blackheads   i) hydraulic chair

_____ used in massage services   j) galvanic machine

_____ an essential barbershop fixture   k) styling brushes

Chapter 7: Anatomy and Physiology

Word Review

abductors
adductors
anabolism
anatomy
angular artery
anterior auricular artery
aorta
aponeurosis
arteries
atrium
auricularis anterior
auricularis posterior
auricularis superior
auriculotemporal nerve
autonomic nervous system
belly of a muscle
blood vascular system
brain
buccal nerve
buccinators
capillaries
carpus
catabolism
cell membrane
cells
central nervous system
cervical cutaneous nerve
cervical nerves
cervical vertebrae
circulatory system
common carotid arteries
corrugator
cranium
cytoplasm
depressor labii inferioris
diaphragm
digestive system
eleventh cranial nerve
endocrine system
epicranius
ethmoid bone
excretory system
external carotid artery
external jugular vein

facial artery
facial bones
fifth cranial nerve
frontal artery
frontal bone
frontalis
greater auricular nerve
greater occipital nerve
gross anatomy
heart
histology
humerous
hyoid bone
indirect division
inferior labial artery
infraorbital artery
infraorbital nerve
infratrochlear nerve
insertion of a muscle
integumentary system
internal carotid artery
internal jugular vein
lacrimal bones
levator anguli oris
levator labii superioris
lungs
lymph
lymph nodes
lymphatic-immune system
mandible bone
mandibular nerve
massester
maxillary bones
mentalis
mental nerve
metabolism
metacarpus
middle temporal artery
mitosis
mixed nerves
motor nerves
muscular system
myology
nasal bones

nasal nerve
nucleus
occipital artery
occipital bone
occipitalis
opponent muscles
orbicularis oculi
orbicularis oris
organs
origin of a muscle
parietal artery
parietal bones
pericardium
peripheral nervous system
phalanges
physiology
plasma
platelets
platysma
posterior auricular artery
posterior auricular nerve
procerus
radius
red blood cells
reflex
reproductive system
respiratory system
risorius
sensory nerves
seventh cranial nerve
skeletal system
smaller occipital nerve
sphenoid bone
spinal cord
sternocleidomastoideus
submental artery
superficial temporal artery
superior labial artery
supraorbital artery
supraorbital nerve
supratrochlear nerve
systems
temporal bones
temporalis

temporal nerve	trapezius	ventricle
thorax	triangularis	white blood cells
tissues	ulna	zygomatic
transverse facial artery	veins	zygomaticus

TOPIC 1: Introduction

A basic knowledge of the structure and functions of the human body assists barbers in the analysis and performance of professional services.

1. These services include _____, _____, _____, and _____ design, _____, _____, and _____ treatments.

2. _____ is the study of the shape and structure of an organism's body and the relationship of one body part to another.

3. _____ is the study of large and easily observable structures of an organism as seen through inspection with the naked eye.

4. _____ is the study of the minute structure of various tissues and organs that make up the entire body of an organism.

5. _____ studies the functions and activities of each body part and the way in which these actions coordinate to form a complete living organism.

TOPIC 2: Cells

The cell is the basic unit of structure and function of all living things.

1. Match the following descriptions with the most correct structure of the cell. Word choices may be used more than once.

_____ most important organelle in the cell

_____ contains food materials for growth

_____ permits soluble substances to leave the cell

_____ located in the center of the cell

_____ encloses the protoplasm

_____ contains less dense protoplasm

_____ contains dense and active protoplasm

_____ permits soluble substances to enter the cell

_____ controls cell activity

_____ facilitates cell division

a) cell membrane

b) nucleus

c) cytoplasm

2. When a cell in the human body reaches maturity, reproduction takes place through
_____.

3. When cells reproduce by dividing into two identical cells called daughter cells, the process is called
_____.

4. Most body cells are capable of growth and _____ during their life cycle.

5. The chemical process through which body cells are nourished and supplied with the energy needed to carry out their many activities is called _____.

6. Constructive metabolism that builds up cellular tissues occurs during _____.

7. The metabolic phase that involves the breaking down of complex compounds within cells into smaller ones is called _____.

8. Anabolism and catabolism are carried out _____ and continually within the cells to facilitate the processes required for life.

TOPIC 3: Tissues

1. Tissues are composed of groups of cells that are similar in shape, size, and structure; each tissue type has a specific _____.

2. Match the following definitions or functions with the most correct word or words. Word choices may be used more than once.

_____ contracts and moves various parts of the body   a) connective tissue

_____ blood and lymph   b) epithelial tissue

_____ binds tissues together   c) liquid tissue

_____ protective covering on body surfaces   d) muscular tissue

_____ carries messages to and from the brain   e) nerve tissue

_____ carries food, waste products, and hormones

_____ examples are bone, cartilage, ligament, tendon, and fat tissue

_____ controls and coordinates all body functions

TOPIC 4: Organs

1. Organs are structures containing two or more _____ that combine to accomplish a specific function.

36

2. Match the following definitions or functions with the correct organ.

_____ excretes water and other waste products

_____ removes toxic products of digestion

_____ control vision

_____ circulates the blood

_____ controls the body

_____ external protective covering of the body

_____ digests food

_____ supply oxygen to the blood

a) brain

b) eyes

c) heart

d) kidneys

e) lungs

f) liver

g) skin

h) stomach and intestines

TOPIC 5: Systems

Systems are groups of organs that act together to perform one or more functions within the body.

1. Each system forms a unit that is designed to perform a specific _____ with the cooperation of other systems.

2. The human body is composed of _____ major systems.

TOPIC 6: Skeletal System

1. The scientific study of bones, their structure, and their functions is called _____.
   The _____ system is the physical foundation of the body and is composed of 206 differently shaped bones.

2. List the primary functions of the skeletal system.

   a) _____

   b) _____

   c) _____

   d) _____

   e) _____

3. The skull consists of 8 bones in the _____ and 14 _____ bones.

4. Label the bones of the skull in the following illustrations. Some of the terms can be used more than once.

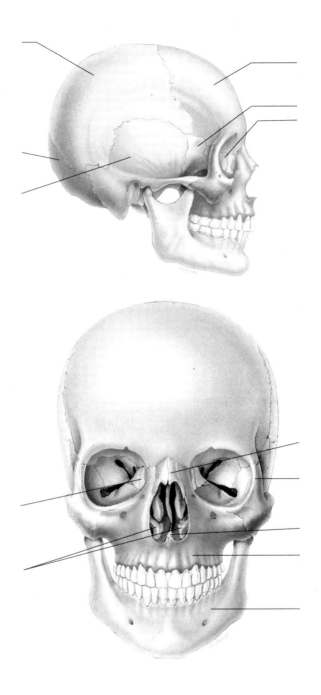

5. Match the following descriptions with the correct bone(s) of the skull.

_____ forms the forehead   a) occipital bone

_____ forms part of the nasal cavities   b) parietal bones

_____ form the sides and top of the cranium   c) frontal bone

_____ joins the bones of the cranium together   d) temporal bones

_____ the hindmost bone of the skull   e) ethmoid bone

_____ form the sides of the head near the ears   f) sphenoid bone

6. Match the following descriptions with the correct bone(s) of the face.

_____ form the bridge of the nose   a) zygomatic bones

_____ small bones at the inner wall of the eye sockets   b) nasal bones

_____ form the prominence of the cheeks   c) mandibles

_____ the upper jawbones   d) lacrimal bones

_____ forms the lower jaw   e) maxillae

7. The U-shaped bone located in the front part of the throat is called the _____ bone.

8. Seven bones that form the top part of the spinal column are called the _____.

9. The _____ consists of the sternum, clavicle, scapula, and 12 pairs of ribs.

10. Match the following descriptions with the correct bone(s) of the shoulders, arms, and hands.

_____ largest bone of the arm   a) metacarpus

_____ innermost and larger bone of the forearm   b) carpus

_____ smaller bone of the forearm   c) humerus

_____ flexible joint composed of eight small bones   d) phalanges

_____ bones of the palm   e) radius

_____ bones in the fingers and toes   f) ulna

TOPIC 7: Muscular System

The muscular system covers, shapes, and supports the skeleton and its function is to help produce movement within the body.

1. _____ is the study of the structure, functions, and diseases of the muscles.

2. The muscular system accounts for _____ to _____ percent of the body's weight.

3. The three types of muscular tissue are _____, _____, and _____.

39

4. A muscle has three parts: origin, belly, and insertion. The _____ of a muscle is more fixed and is attached to bones or other muscles; the _____ is the middle part of the muscle; the _____ is the more movable attachment.

5. Pressure used in massage is usually directed from the _____ to the _____ of the muscle.

6. List the methods that may be used to stimulate muscular tissues.

a) _____

b) _____

c) _____

d) _____

e) _____

f) _____

g) _____

7. Barbers must be concerned with the _____ muscles of the head, face, and neck.

8. Label the muscles of the head, face, and neck in the following illustration.

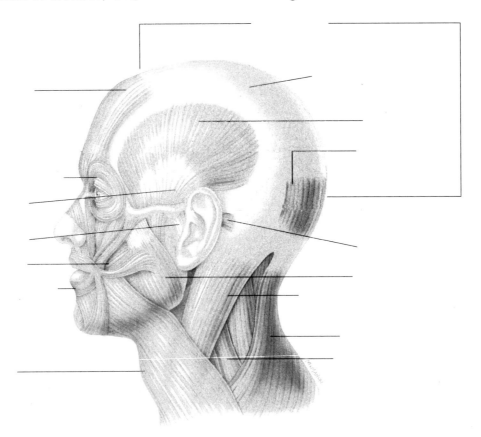

9. Label the muscles of the face in the following illustration.

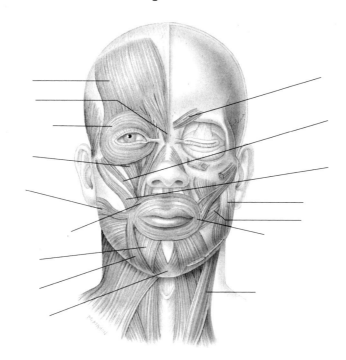

10. Match the following descriptions or functions with the correct muscles of the scalp, face, and neck.

_____ muscle that covers the top of the skull

_____ draws the scalp backward

_____ connects the occipitalis and the frontalis

_____ draws the scalp forward

_____ draws the eyebrows down and in

_____ surrounds the eye socket

_____ covers the top of the nose

_____ surrounds the upper lip

_____ compresses the cheeks

_____ depresses the lower lip

_____ pushes up the lower lip

_____ raises the angle of the mouth

_____ a flat band around the upper and lower lips

_____ draws the corner of the mouth out and back

_____ elevates the lip

_____ draws down the corner of the mouth

_____ draws the ear backward

_____ draws the ear upward

a) frontalis

b) orbicularis oculi

c) corrugator

d) procerus

e) epicranius

f) occipitalis

g) buccinator

h) aponeurosis

i) triangularis

j) zygomaticus

k) risorius

l) orbicularis oris

m) levator labii superioris

n) depressor labii inferioris

o) levator anguli oris

p) auricularis superior

q) mentalis

r) auricularis posterior

41

_____ draws the ear forward

_____ chewing muscles

_____ depresses the lower jaw and lip

_____ bends and rotates the head

_____ allows shoulder movement

_____ separates fingers

_____ draws the fingers together

_____ brings the thumb toward the fingers

s) masseter and temporalis

t) auricularis anterior

u) platysma

v) abductors

w) sternocleidomastoideus

x) adductors

y) opponent

z) trapezius

TOPIC 8: Nervous System

The nervous system is one of the most important systems of the body. It controls and coordinates the functions of all the other systems and makes them work harmoniously and efficiently.

1. The study of the structure, function, and pathology of the nervous system is called

   _____.

2. An understanding of how nerves work helps barbers to perform _____ services associated with shampoos, scalp treatments, and facials.

3. The cerebrospinal, or _____ system, consists of the brain, cranial nerves, spinal cord, and spinal nerves. It controls consciousness and all mental activities, voluntary functions of the five senses, voluntary muscle actions, body movements, and _____ _____.

4. The _____ nervous system is made up of sensory and motor nerve fibers that extend from the brain and spinal cord to all parts of the body. Their function is to carry impulses, or messages, to and from the _____ nervous system.

5. The _____, or sympathetic, nervous system is important in the operation of internal body functions such as breathing, circulation, digestion, and glandular activities. Its main purpose is to _____ these internal operations, keeping them in balance and working properly.

6. Stimulation to the nerves causes muscles to contract and expand. List the ways in which nerve stimulation may be accomplished.

   a) _____

   b) _____

   c) _____

   d) _____

   e) _____

   f) _____

7. There are three types of nerves: _____ nerves carry impulses or messages from sense organs to the brain; _____ nerves carry impulses from the brain to the muscles; and _____ nerves contain both sensory and motor fibers and have the ability to send and receive messages.

8. A _____ is an automatic nerve reaction to a stimulus.

There are 12 pairs of cranial nerves. The most important cranial nerves for barbers to know when massaging the head, face, and neck are the fifth cranial, seventh cranial, eleventh cranial, and cervical nerves, which originate in the spinal column.

9. Match the following descriptions or functions with the correct nerve. Terms may be used more than once.

A. Fifth Cranial Nerve

_____ motor nerve of chewing muscles	a) supraorbital
_____ also known as the fifth cranial nerve	b) supratrochlear
_____ affects the membrane and skin of the nose	c) nasal
_____ affects skin between the eyes and upper sides of the nose	d) zygomatic
_____ affects the skin of the temples	e) trifacial
_____ affects the external ear	f) mental
_____ affects the skin of the lower lip and chin	g) infraorbital
_____ affects the skin of the lower eyelids	h) auriculotemporal
_____ affects the skin of the forehead and scalp	i) infratrochlear
_____ affects the point and lower sides of the nose	

B. Seventh Cranial Nerve

_____ chief motor nerve of the face	a) posterior auricular
_____ affects muscles of the temples	b) facial nerve
_____ affects muscles of the chin and lower lip	c) temporal
_____ affects muscles of the mouth	d) zygomatic
_____ also known as the seventh cranial nerve	e) buccal
_____ affects muscles behind the ears	f) mandibular
_____ affects muscles of the upper cheek areas	g) cervical
_____ controls all the muscles used for facial expression	
_____ affects the sides of the neck	
_____ affects muscles of the eyebrows and eyelids	

C. Eleventh Cranial Nerve

_____ affects the scalp in back to the top of the head	a) greater auricular
_____ affects the scalp at the base of the skull	b) cutaneous colli
_____ affects area in front and back of the ears	c) greater occipital
_____ affects the front and sides of the neck	d) smaller or lesser occipital

TOPIC 9: Circulatory System

The circulatory system, also referred to as the cardiovascular or vascular system, controls the steady circulation of the blood and is made up of two divisions.

1. The _____ system consists of the heart, arteries, capillaries, and veins for the circulation and distribution of blood throughout the body.

2. The _____ system aids the blood vascular system in the transportation of fluids.

3. The heart is a muscular, conical organ about the size of a closed fist that keeps the blood moving within the circulatory system. The heart weighs approximately _____ ounces and the normal heartbeat of an adult is _____ to _____ beats a minute.

4. The interior of the heart contains four chambers and four valves. The _____ chambers are the right atrium and left atrium and the _____ chambers are the right ventricle and left ventricle. _____ allow the blood to flow in only one direction.

5. Blood vessels are tube-like structures that include _____, _____, and _____. They transport blood to and from the heart and to various body tissues.

6. _____ are thick-walled, muscular, elastic tubes that carry pure blood from the heart to the capillaries.

7. Capillaries are minute, thin-walled blood vessels that connect smaller arteries with _____.

8. _____ are thin-walled vessels that contain valves to prevent back-flow. They carry deoxygenated blood from the capillaries back to the heart.

9. _____ circulation is the blood circulation that goes from the heart to the lungs to be purified, and then returns to the heart.

10. _____ circulation is the blood circulation from the heart throughout the body and back again to the heart.

11. The average adult has 8 to 10 _____ of blood.

The blood is composed of one-third red and white corpuscles and blood platelets, and two-thirds plasma.

12. _____ blood cells are produced in the bone marrow, and their function is to carry _____ to the body cells.

13. _____ blood cells destroy disease-causing germs.

14. _____ contribute to the blood-clotting process that stops bleeding.

15. _____ is the fluid part of the blood in which blood cell platelets flow, and its main function is to carry food and secretions to the cells and to take carbon dioxide.

16. List the chief functions of the blood.

a) _____

b) _____

_____

c) _____

d) _____

e) _____

TOPIC 10: Lymphatic-Immune System

1. The _____ system consists of lymph, _____, the thymus gland, spleen, and lymph vessels, and acts as an aid to the blood system.

2. Lymph is a colorless, watery fluid derived from _____.

3. List the chief functions of the lymphatic-immune system.

a) _____

b) _____

c) _____

TOPIC 11: Arteries of the Head, Face, and Neck

1. The main sources of the _____ supply to the head, face, and neck are the arteries.

2. Blood is supplied to the brain, eye sockets, eyelids, and forehead through the _____ carotid artery. The _____ carotid artery supplies blood to the front parts of the head, face, and neck.

3. Label the arteries of the head, face, and neck in the following illustration.

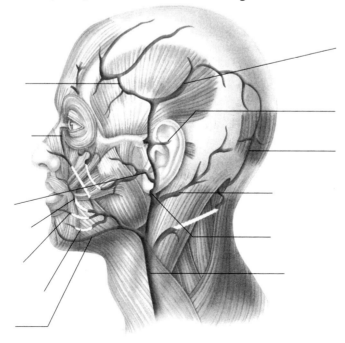

4. Match the following descriptions or functions with the correct facial artery.

_____ supplies the upper lip and septum   a) frontal artery

_____ supplies the chin and lower lip   b) anterior auricular artery

_____ supplies the sides of the nose   c) parietal artery

_____ supplies the lower lip   d) middle temporal artery

_____ supplies the forehead   e) transverse facial artery

_____ supplies the crown and sides of the head   f) occipital artery

_____ supplies the masseter   g) posterior auricular artery

_____ supplies the temples and eyelids   h) submental artery

_____ supplies the anterior part of the ear   i) facial artery

_____ supplies the scalp and back of the head to the crown   j) inferior labial artery

_____ supplies the scalp behind and above the ear   k) superficial temporal artery

_____ supplies blood to the lower region of the face   l) angular artery

_____ a continuation of the external carotid artery   m) superior labial artery

5. The blood returns to the heart from the head, face, and neck through the _____
   jugular and _____ jugular veins.

TOPIC 12: Other Systems

1. The _____ system consists of a group of specialized glands that affect the growth, development, sexual activities, and health of the entire body.

2. _____ are specialized organs that vary in size and function. They have the ability to remove certain elements from the _____ and to convert them into new compounds.

3. _____ glands, also known as _____ glands, have canals that lead from the gland to a particular part of the body. _____ and _____ glands are examples of exocrine glands.

4. _____ glands are ductless glands that release secretions called hormones directly into the bloodstream where they stimulate functional activity or secretion in other parts of the body.

5. The digestive system is responsible for changing food into nutrients and waste. The entire digestive process takes about _____ to complete.

6. The excretory system purifies the body by eliminating waste matter. The organs that play a crucial role in the process are the _____, _____, _____, large _____, and _____.

7. The _____ system enables breathing and consists of the lungs and air passages.

8. The _____ inhale oxygen and exchange it for carbon dioxide during one breathing cycle.

9. The _____ is a muscular partition that separates the thorax from the abdominal region and helps control breathing.

10. _____ breathing is healthier than _____ breathing.

11. _____ breathing means deep breathing, which creates the greatest exchange of gases.

12. The _____ system consists of the skin and its appendages, such as sweat glands and oil glands, hair, nails, and sensory receptors. The _____ is the body's largest organ.

Chapter 8: Chemistry

Word Review

acid-balanced shampoos	emulsions	pH scale
acids	inorganic chemistry	physical change
alkalis	instant conditioners	physical mixture
atoms	ion	physical properties
balancing shampoos	ionization	protein conditioners
bases	leave-in conditioners	pure substance
bluing rinses	liquid-dry shampoos	redox
chemical change	matter	reduction
chemical properties	medicated rinses	rinses
chemistry	medicated shampoos	salts
clarifying shampoos	moisturizing conditioners	scalp conditioners
color-enhancing shampoos	moisturizing shampoos	shampoo
compound molecules	molecule	surfactants
compounds	organic chemistry	suspensions
conditioners	organic shampoos	synthetic polymer conditioners
deep-conditioning treatments	oxidation	tonic
dry or powder shampoos	oxides	
element	pH	

TOPIC 1: Introduction

1. One of the most important uses of chemicals in the barbershop is the application of disinfectant and cleaning solutions to maintain an effective program of _____.

2. Chemicals are also involved in the performance of services when a _____ change to the structure of the hair is desired.

TOPIC 2: Basic Chemistry

Chemistry is the science that deals with the composition, structure, and properties of matter and how matter changes under different chemical conditions.

1. Organic chemistry is the study of substances that contain _____.

2. The word _____ applies to all living things and those things that were once alive.

3. Most organic substances will _____.

4. _____ chemistry is the study of substances that do not contain carbon.

5. Some examples of inorganic substances are: _____

   _____.

6. Matter is anything that occupies space and has physical and chemical properties. It exists in the states of _____, _____, and _____.

7. Visible light and color are forms of _____ and therefore are not matter. Matter exists in the forms of _____, _____, and _____.

8. _____ are pure chemical substances that cannot be separated into simpler substances by chemical means. Chemical elements are the basic _____ that make up all matter, and each one has its own kind of atom. Each element is given a letter symbol. One such example is _____.

9. Atoms are the basic _____ of all matter.

10. An _____ is the smallest part of an element that retains the characteristics of that element.

11. A molecule is formed when two or more atoms are joined by a chemical bond. _____ molecules are chemical combinations of two or more atoms of the same element; an example is _____. _____ molecules are chemical combinations of two or more atoms of different elements; an example is _____.

12. All matter exists in one of three different physical forms: solid, liquid, or gas. Match the following examples with the correct form of matter.

    _____ water   a) solid

    _____ ice   b) liquid

    _____ steam   c) gas

13. The two different types of properties are _____ and _____.

14. Characteristics that can be determined without a chemical reaction and without a chemical change in the identity of the substance indicate _____ properties.

15. Characteristics that can only be determined with a chemical reaction and that cause a chemical change in the identity of the substance indicate _____ properties.

16. Identify the following characteristics with a "P" or a "C" as representing physical or chemical properties.

    _____ color

    _____ rusting iron

    _____ melting point

    _____ odor

    _____ density

    _____ wood burning to ash

17. A pure substance is matter that has a fixed chemical composition, definite proportions, and distinct properties; _____ and _____ are examples of pure substances.

18. Elemental molecules contain two or more atoms of the _____ element that unite _____.

19. Chemical compounds are combinations of two or more atoms of different elements that unite _____ as a result of a chemical _____.

20. Identify the following descriptions as defining bases, acids, oxides, or salts.

    _____ compounds of hydrogen, a non-metal such as nitrogen and, sometimes, oxygen

    _____ compounds of hydrogen, a metal, and oxygen

    _____ compounds formed by the reaction of acids and bases

    _____ compounds of any element combined with oxygen

    _____ example: one part carbon and two parts oxygen

    _____ turn blue litmus paper red

    _____ also known as alkalis

    _____ example: sodium and chloride

    _____ example: magnesium, sulphur, hydrogen, and oxygen

    _____ turn red litmus paper blue

    _____ example: hydrogen, sulphur, and oxygen

    _____ example: sodium, oxygen, and hydrogen

21. A physical mixture is a combination of two more substances united physically in any proportion without a fixed composition; pure _____ and _____ are examples of physical mixtures.

TOPIC 3: Chemistry of Water

A. Water (H_2O) is the most abundant and important of all chemicals, composing about 75 percent of the earth's surface and about 65 percent of the human body.

   1. Water is the universal _____.

   2. Water is purified through _____, _____, or _____.

   3. Boiling water at _____ degrees Fahrenheit destroys most microbes and makes it suitable for drinking.

   4. Examples of soft water are _____ and chemically _____ water.

   5. Hard water contains mineral substances that inhibit the formation of soap _____.

50

B. The pH Scale: The letters *pH* denote potential hydrogen.

  1. The term *pH* means the relative degree of _____ or _____ of a substance.

  2. The pH scale measures the _____ of hydrogen ions in acidic and alkaline solutions.

  3. In pure water, some of the water molecules ionize naturally into hydrogen ions and hydroxide ions. The hydrogen ion is _____ and the hydroxide ion is _____.

  5. The pH values are arranged on a scale ranging from 0 to 14. A pH of _____ indicates a neutral solution, below 7 indicates an _____ solution, and above 7 indicates an _____ solution.

  6. A change of one whole number on the pH scale represents a _____ change in pH.

  7. Pure water can cause the hair to swell up to _____ percent.

C. Acids and Alkalis

  1. Identify the following solutions as being acidic, alkaline, or neutral.

     _____ hair and skin

     _____ hydrogen peroxide

     _____ distilled water

     _____ blood

     _____ neutral permanent waves

     _____ vinegar

     _____ soaps

     _____ lemon juice

     _____ depilatories

     _____ relaxers

     _____ semipermanent color

     _____ neutralizers

     _____ cold wave lotion

     _____ conditioners

     _____ tints

  2. _____ contract and harden the hair and tighten the skin.

  3. _____ soften and swell the hair.

  4. When acids and alkalis are mixed together in equal proportions, they _____ each other to form water and a salt.

D. Oxidation-Reduction Reactions

1. _____ is a chemical reaction that combines an element or compound with oxygen to produce an oxide.

2. Oxidizing agents are substances that release oxygen. When oxygen is combined with a substance, the substance is _____ . When oxygen is removed from a substance, the substance is _____ .

3. Oxidation and reduction always occur simultaneously; they are referred to as _____ reactions. In these reactions, the oxidizer is always _____ and the reducing agent is always _____ .

4. Oxidation also results from the _____ of hydrogen, and reduction is the result of the _____ of hydrogen.

5. The result of mixing hydrogen peroxide with a haircoloring product is an example of _____ . The loss of oxygen in the hydrogen peroxide during the process is an example of _____ .

TOPIC 4: Cosmetic Chemistry

1. The physical and chemical classifications of cosmetics used in the barbershop are

_____ .

2. Match the following descriptions with the most correct term.

_____ mixtures that do not separate upon standing

_____ uniform mixtures of insoluble substances

_____ uniform mixtures of two or more substances

_____ two immiscible liquids held together by an agent

_____ substances that allow oil and water to mix or emulsify

_____ compounds made of oils or fats and alkaline substances

_____ semi-solid mixes of organic substances and a medicinal agent

a) suspensions

b) ointments

c) solutions

d) powders

e) emulsions

f) surfactants

g) soaps

TOPIC 5: Cosmetic Preparations

A. Shampoos

1. Most shampoo products are _____ .

2. The purpose of a shampoo product and service is to _____ the scalp and hair.

3. To be effective, a shampoo product should:

a) _____

b) _____

c) _____

d) _____

6. Shampoo product selection should be based on the _____.

7. Shampoos are available for _____, _____,
_____, coarse, limp or _____ hair.

8. The acidity or alkalinity of a shampoo product is important because

_____.

9. _____ solutions shrink, constrict, and harden the cuticle scales of the hair shaft.

10. _____ solutions soften, swell, and expand the hair shaft cuticle scales.

11. Shampoo products usually range between _____ and _____
on the pH scale.

12. The normal pH range for hair and skin is _____ to _____.

13. Shampoos consist of two main ingredients: _____ and surfactants.

14. Shampoo molecules are composed of a _____ and a _____.

15. The _____ of the shampoo _____ molecule attracts dirt,
grease, debris, and oil, but it repels water.

16. The _____ of the shampoo molecule attracts water but repels dirt.

17. Next to water, surfactants are the second most common ingredient found in shampoos;
surfactants can take the form of _____, _____, or
_____ agents.

18. The base surfactant or combination of surfactants determines the _____ of a
shampoo; however, most manufacturers use detergents from more than one group.

19. Label the characteristics and descriptions with the appropriate type of surfactant (anionic,
cationic, nonionic, or ampholyte).

_____ most commonly used detergents

_____ valued for their versatility

_____ behave as an anionic or a cationic based on pH

_____ sodium lauryl sulfate is an example

_____ consist mostly of quats

_____ used in baby shampoos

_____ low incidence of irritation to human tissues

_____ strong, rich, foaming detergent

_____ have some antibacterial action

_____ sodium laureth sulfate is an example

_____ stable and resist shrinkage

_____ may be used in dandruff shampoos

_____ cocamide is an example

_____ possess germicidal properties

20. Liquid shampoos are available in _____ or _____ forms.

21. _____ shampoos are used for cleansing the scalp and hair when the client is prevented by illness from having a regular shampoo.

22. _____ or _____ shampoos are used when the client's health will not permit a _____ shampoo. These shampoos may contain _____ powder and should never be used prior to a _____ service.

23. _____ shampoos are balanced to the pH level of hair and skin, are mild, and prevent the stripping of hair color from the hair; they are also a good choice for normal, _____, and _____ hair.

24. Moisturizing or _____ shampoos are usually mild, cream shampoos that contain moisturizing agents.

25. _____ either "lock in" the moisturizing properties of the product or draw moisture into the hair, and do not remove artificial _____ from the hair.

26. Shampoos designed to cut through product or hard-water mineral buildup are called _____ shampoos.

27. _____ shampoos are designed for oily hair and scalp.

28. _____ shampoos contain a medicinal agent such as sulfur, tar, or another antiseptic agent; _____ medicated shampoos contain special chemicals or drugs that are effective in reducing dandruff and must be used only by _____.

29. Organic shampoos are usually _____.

30. _____ shampoos are created by combining the surfactant with basic colors and are used to brighten, add slight color, or eliminate unwanted color tones.

B. Conditioners

1. Conditioners can be either _____ or _____ conditioners.

2. Hair conditioners usually _____ the hair; scalp conditioners are used for maintenance or to treat conditions requiring a _____ product.

3. Conditioners can deposit _____ or _____ in the hair.

4. The typical pH range of conditioners is _____ to _____ on the pH scale.

5. Conditioners are _____ remedies for hair that feels dry or is damaged.

6. Excessive use or the wrong type of conditioner can lead to product _____ that makes the hair feel heavy and oily.

7. As with shampoo products, barbers need to be able to select the _____ conditioning product for their clients.

8. The three basics types of conditioners are _____, _____, and _____.

9. _____ conditioners are applied to the hair following a shampoo and are rinsed out after _____; finishing conditioners, detangling conditioners, and _____ are examples of instant conditioners.

10. _____ conditioners are usually heavier than instant conditioners and have an application time of _____ ; they may require heat for deeper penetration.

11. _____ conditioners have the ability to pass through the cuticle to the cortex where _____ has been lost from the hair, and can improve texture, _____ , and help to increase elasticity in the hair.

12. _____ are chemical mixtures of concentrated protein in the heavy cream base of a moisturizer and are used when equal degrees of moisturization and protein deposit is desired.

13. _____ conditioners are special formulations that are designed for use on badly damaged hair to prevent further damage.

14. _____ conditioners are products that _____ be rinsed out of the hair and can be used to help equalize _____ .

15. Some _____ are cream-based products with moisturizers and emollients used to soften the scalp and improve its health.

16. _____ scalp tonics help to remove oil accumulation on the scalp and may be used after a scalp treatment.

C. Rinses

1. A hair _____ is an agent used to cleanse or condition the hair and scalp, bring out the luster of the hair, or add highlights.

2. _____ rinses are used to wet and rinse the hair during the shampoo service.

3. _____ rinses are formulated to control minor dandruff and scalp conditions.

4. _____ rinses are preparations that contain a blue base color to counteract yellowish or dull gray tones in the hair; these rinses also neutralize the hair to silvery gray or white tones.

D. Tonics

1. It is important for barbers to understand the ingredients, specific _____ , and uses of each type of hair tonic.

2. Hair tonics are available in _____ , _____ , _____ , and _____ formulations.

3. Review the following hair tonic descriptions and match each with the correct type. Choices may be used more than once.

_____ contains antiseptic and alcohol

_____ contains antiseptic solution and grooming ingredients

_____ contains alcohol and oil

_____ acts as a mild astringent

_____ contains lanolin and mineral oils

a) non-alcoholic tonic

b) alcohol-based tonic

c) cream or emulsion tonic

d) oil-mixture tonic

4. For maximum benefit, tonic applications should include a _____ .

E. Other Cosmetic Preparations

1. Astringents may have an alcohol content of up to 35 percent. They cause
    _____ of the skin tissues.

2. _____ creams are used during facials and shaves and have the ability to
    dissolve _____ substances.

3. Cleansing _____ serve the same purposes as cleansing creams but are of a
    lighter consistency and are usually water-based _____.

4. Preparations used for the temporary removal of superfluous hair by dissolving it at the skin
    line are called _____.

5. _____ remove hair by pulling it out of the follicle through the use of waxes.

6. _____ have the lowest alcohol content of the tonic lotions and are designed
    for dry, mature, and sensitive skin types.

7. _____, such as pomades, give shine and manageability to dry or curly hair.

9. _____ is used to hold the finished hairstyle in place.

10. _____ and _____ are available for deep cleansing, pore
    reduction, tightening, firming, moisturizing, and wrinkle reduction.

11. _____ creams are used to help the hands to glide over the skin during
    a facial.

12. _____ lotions are available by prescription for skin problems such as acne
    or rashes.

13. _____ creams are designed to treat dryness and contain _____.

14. Scalp lotions and ointments usually contain _____ agents for correction of a
    scalp condition, such as itching or flakiness.

15. Two styling aids that may contain polymers, moisturizers, and/or humectants are
    _____ and _____.

16. _____ lotions are designed to protect the skin from the harmful ultraviolet
    rays of the sun.

17. Skin _____ usually have an alcohol content of 4 to 15 percent and are
    designed for use on normal and combination skin types.

18. The alcohols most often used in the barbershop are _____ alcohol and
    _____ alcohol.

19. Styptic powder or liquid is made from _____.

20. _____ is a solution of alcohol, water, and powder ground from certain leaves
    and twigs that works as an astringent and skin freshener.

21. The _____ is a public health organization that sets standards for
    food ingredients, health-care products, and drugs sold or manufactured in the United States
    and used by the public.

Date: _____

Rating: _____

Text Pages 202–217

Chapter 9: Electricity and Light Therapy

Word Review

alternating current	electric current	polarity
amp (ampere)	electrode	rectifier
anaphoresis	electrotherapy	rheostat
anode	faradic current	sinusoidal current
cataphoresis	fuse	Tesla high-frequency
cathode	galvanic current	current
circuit breaker	ground fault circuit interrupter	ultraviolet light
complete circuit	infrared rays	visible light
conductor	insulator	volt
converter	iontophoresis	watt
desincrustation	modalities	wavelength
direct current	ohm	

TOPIC 1: Introduction

Electricity is a valuable tool for barbers, provided it is used carefully and intelligently.

1. Electricity is a form of energy that produces _____, _____, or _____ effects while in motion.

2. An _____ current is the flow of electricity along a conductor.

3. Match the following definitions with the correct word or words. Choices may be combined (e.g., "a and b") or used more than once.

_____ a substance that does not easily transmit electricity   a) conductor

_____ path of an electric current from the source and back again   b) insulator

_____ used for controlling the current in a circuit   c) nonconductor

_____ rubber or silk coverings   d) electric wire

_____ changes direct current to alternating current   e) complete circuit

_____ twisted metal threads that act as a conductor   f) converter

_____ any substance or material that conducts electricity   g) rheostat

_____ an adjustable resistor   h) rectifier

_____ changes alternating current to direct current

_____ also known as insulator

_____ most metals, carbon, the human body, and watery solutions

57

4. The type of current that travels in one direction only and produces a chemical reaction is called _____ current.

5. The type of current that produces a mechanical action by flowing first in one direction and then the other is an _____ current.

6. The electrical pressure that pushes the flow of electrons forward through a conductor is called _____ and is measured in a unit called a _____ .

7. The standard unit for measuring the strength of an electric current is an _____ or _____ .

8. The current for facial and scalp treatments is measured in _____ , or one one-thousandth of an _____ .

9. An _____ is a unit that measures the resistance of an electrical current.

10. A _____ measures how much electric energy is being used in one second.

11. A safety device that prevents the overheating of electrical wires by preventing excessive current from passing through a circuit is called a _____ .

12. A _____ is a switch that automatically interrupts or shuts off an electric circuit at the first indication of an overload.

13. A life-saving device that senses imbalances within an electric circuit is a _____ .

14. A third, circular prong on some electrical plugs provides an additional _____ .

15. All electrical equipment should be inspected regularly to help eliminate accidental shocks, fires, and burns. Review the electrical equipment safety reminders found in the textbook, and fill in the blanks to complete the following sentences.

   a) All electrical appliances should be _____ certified.

   b) Study the _____ before using any electrical equipment.

   c) _____ appliances when not in use.

   d) Keep all wires, plugs, and equipment in good repair and _____ all electrical equipment frequently.

   e) Do not overload _____ .

   f) Avoid _____ electrical cords.

   g) When using electrical equipment, _____ the _____ at all times.

   h) Do not touch any _____ while using an electrical appliance.

   i) Do not handle electrical equipment with _____ .

j) Do not allow the client to touch any _____ surfaces while being treated with electrical equipment.

k) Do not _____ the _____ while a client is connected to an electrical device.

l) Do not attempt to clean around an electric outlet while equipment is _____ in.

m) Do not touch two metallic objects at the same time if either is connected to an

_____ .

n) Do not step on or set objects on electrical _____ .

o) Do not allow electrical cords to become twisted or bent because the wires inside the cord will _____ and the _____ will wear away from the wires.

p) Disconnect the appliance by pulling on the _____ , not the _____ .

q) Do not _____ electrical appliances unless you are qualified to do so.

TOPIC 2: Electrotherapy

Electronic facial and scalp treatments are commonly referred to as electrotherapy.

1. The different types of currents used in electrotherapy treatments are called _____ .

2. An _____ is an applicator used to direct the electric current from the machine to the client's skin.

3. Electrodes are usually made of _____ , _____ , or _____ .

4. _____ indicates the negative or positive pole of an electric current.

5. The positive pole is called an _____ and is usually _____ in color.

6. The negative electrode is called a _____ and is usually _____ in color.

7. Anodes may also be marked with a _____ or _____ sign.

8. Cathodes may also be marked with a _____ or _____ sign.

9. _____ are the currents used in electronic facial and scalp treatments. The four main modalities used in barbering are the _____ , _____ , _____ , and _____ currents.

59

10. Review the following definitions and electrotherapy terms. Match the definitions with the correct word or term. Choices may be combined (e.g., "a and b") or used more than once.

_____ the introduction of ions

_____ alternating currents producing mechanical reaction

_____ used to facilitate deep pore cleansing

_____ has a high rate of oscillation that produces heat

_____ does not cause muscular contractions

_____ causes muscular contractions

_____ most commonly used modality

_____ emulsifies sebum and waste in pores

_____ forces liquids into tissues from negative to positive poles

_____ effects are either stimulating or soothing

_____ forces acidic substances into tissues from positive to negative

a) desincrustation

b) cataphoresis

c) anaphoresis

d) Tesla high-frequency current

e) faradic current

f) sinusoidal current

g) galvanic current

h) iontophoresis

TOPIC 3: Light Therapy

Light therapy, also known as phototherapy, refers to the use of light waves to effect treatments. This is accomplished through the use of therapeutic lamps.

1. Different light rays will produce _____, _____ or _____ reactions.

2. _____ light is electromagnetic radiation—also called _____—that we can see.

3. The distance between two successive peaks of radiant energy is called the _____. Short wavelengths have a higher frequency. Why is this? _____ _____.

4. Visible light is the part of the electromagnetic spectrum that we can see and makes up _____ of natural sunlight.

5. _____ rays and _____ rays are invisible because their wavelengths are beyond the visible spectrum of light. Invisible rays make up _____ natural sunlight.

6. Barbers are concerned with the rays that produce _____ and those that produce _____ and _____ reactions.

7. Review the following characteristics of therapy bulbs. Match the characteristics with the correct word or term. Choices may be used more than once.

_____ combination light

_____ produces the most heat

_____ contains all the visible rays

_____ contains few heat rays

_____ used on bare, clean skin only

_____ penetrates the deepest

_____ used on dry skin

_____ provides germicidal and chemical benefits

_____ aids penetration of lanolin creams into the skin

_____ relieves pain in congested areas

_____ primary light sources used for scalp and facial treatments

a) visible light rays

b) red light

c) blue light

d) white light

8. Ultraviolet rays, also known as _____ rays or _____ rays, make up _____ of natural sunlight.

9. UV rays have short wavelengths, produce _____ effects, kill _____, and are the least penetrating rays.

10. Three types of ultraviolet lamps are the glass bulb, the _____ quartz, and the _____ quartz.

11. The glass bulb lamp is used mainly for _____ or _____ purposes.

12. The hot quartz lamp is an _____ lamp suitable for tanning, tonic, cosmetic, or germicidal purposes.

13. The cold quartz lamp is used primarily in _____.

14. The farther away from the visible light spectrum, the shorter and _____ penetrating the ultraviolet rays.

15. Review the following characteristics of ultraviolet rays and match the characteristics with the correct category of ultraviolet (UV) rays. Choices may be used more than once.

_____ the therapeutic rays

_____ the tonic UV rays

_____ the most germicidal UV rays

_____ used in tanning booths

_____ most penetrating UV rays

_____ cause the most burning to the skin

_____ longest of all the UV rays

_____ destructive to bacteria

a) UVA rays

b) UVB rays

c) UVC rays

16. Ultraviolet rays can be used to treat acne, _____, _____, and dandruff conditions.

17. Ultraviolet rays are applied with a lamp at a distance of _____" to _____" from the skin. Exposure time should start with a short exposure of _____ to _____ minutes and gradually increase to _____ or _____ minutes.

18. Beyond the red rays of the spectrum are the _____ rays. They are pure heat rays that comprise about _____ of sunshine.

19. Infrared rays are long and have the _____ penetration. Infrared rays produce the most _____.

20. Infrared ray treatments will _____ and relax the skin, increase _____ and metabolism, and create _____ changes in the skin.

21. The infrared lamp should be operated at an average distance of _____" from the skin.

22. The length of exposure for infrared treatments should not exceed _____ minutes.

23. To prevent overexposure, it is important to _____ the path of the rays every few seconds.

Chapter 10: Properties and Disorders of the Skin

Word Review

acne	excoriation	sebaceous glands
adipose tissue	fissure	seborrhea
albinism	herpes simplex	sebum
anhidrosis	hyperhidrosis	secretory nerve fibers
anthrax	hypertrophy	sensory nerve fibers
asteatosis	ivy dermatitis	squamous cell carcinoma
basal cell carcinoma	keloid	stain
blackhead	keratoma	steatoma
bromhidrosis	lentigines	strata
bulla	lesion	stratum corneum
chloasma	leukoderma	stratum germinativum
cicatrix	macule	stratum granulosum
collagen	malignant melanoma	stratum lucidum
comedone	melanin	stratum spinosm
corium	milia	subcutaneous tissue
crust	miliaria rubra	sudoriferous glands
cuticle	mole	symptoms
cutis	motor nerve fibers	tan
cyst	nevus	true skin
derma	papillary layer	tubercule
dermatitis	papule	tumor
dermatitis venenata	psoriasis	ulcer
dermatology	pustule	verruca
dermis	reticular layer	vesicle
eczema	rosacea	vitiligo
elastin	scale	wheal
epidermis	scarf skin	whitehead

TOPIC 1: Introduction

Dermatology is the scientific study of the histology of the skin: its nature, structure, functions, diseases, and treatment. A study of the skin and scalp is important to barbers because it forms the basis for effective skin and scalp treatment programs.

1. The skin is the _____ organ of the body.

2. Healthy skin is slightly _____, soft, elastic, and flexible, with a smooth, fine-grained texture.

3. Skin varies in thickness and is thinnest on the _____ and thickest on the _____ of the hands and _____ of the feet.

4. The skin of the scalp is similar to skin elsewhere on the human body, but the scalp has larger and _____ hair follicles to accommodate the longer hair on the head.

5. The appendages of the skin are _____, _____, _____ glands, and _____ glands.

6. The skin is constructed of two primary divisions: the _____ and the _____.

TOPIC 2: Epidermis

The epidermis is the outermost, protective layer of the skin.

1. The epidermis also known as the _____ or _____ skin.

2. The epidermis is the _____ layer of the skin and contains no _____, but has many small _____ endings.

3. The layers of the epidermis are the stratum _____, stratum _____, stratum _____, stratum _____ and the stratum _____.

4. Review the following characteristics of the layers of the epidermis, then match the descriptions with the correct stratum or layer.

_____ lies beneath the stratum corneum	a) stratum corneum
_____ also known as the stratum mucosum	b) stratum lucidum
_____ consists of granular cells	c) stratum granulosum
_____ responsible for epidermal growth	d) stratum germinativum
_____ outermost epidermal layer	e) stratum spinosum

_____ the clear layer

_____ the spiny layer

_____ also known as scarf skin

_____ the horny layer

_____ deepest epidermal layer

_____ the granular layer

_____ also known as the basal layer

_____ contains keratin

_____ contains melanin

_____ consists of transparent cells

_____ replaces cells shed from the stratum corneum

_____ protects against UV rays

64

TOPIC 3: Dermis

The dermis is the inner layer of the skin, situated beneath the epidermis.

1. The dermis is also known as the _____, _____, _____, or _____ skin.

2. The dermis is about _____ times thicker than the epidermis and consists of _____ tissue.

3. The dermis consists of the _____ and _____ layers.

4. The _____ layer lies directly beneath the epidermis. It contains projections of elastic tissue called _____, looped _____, _____ endings, and _____.

5. The _____ layer is the deeper dermal layer and supplies the skin with oxygen and nutrients. The structures within this layer are _____ cells, _____ glands, _____, _____, _____ glands, _____ muscles, and _____ glands.

6. The layer of fatty tissue found below the dermis is called _____ or _____. This tissue varies in thickness according to age, gender, and general health; some specialists consider it a continuation of the _____.

7. Subcutaneous tissue gives smoothness and contour to the body, contains _____ for use as energy, and acts as a _____ for the outer skin.

8. Identify and label the following illustration with the layers and structures of the skin.

9. How is the skin nourished? _____

10. One-half to two-thirds of the body's _____ supply is distributed to the skin.

TOPIC 4: Nerves of the Skin

1. The skin contains many nerve fiber endings. These are classified as _____ nerve fibers, _____ nerve fibers, and _____ nerve fibers.

2. Use either *motor, sensory*, or *secretory* to correctly identify the type of nerve fiber associated with the following nerve characteristics.

   _____ react to heat and cold

   _____ are distributed to sweat glands

   _____ are distributed to arrector pili muscles

   _____ regulate the flow of sebum

   _____ react to touch, pressure, and pain

   _____ regulate the excretion of perspiration

   _____ cause goose bumps

   _____ send messages to the brain

3. Nerve endings that provide the body with the sense of touch are located in the _____ layer of the _____.

4. Nerve endings are most abundant in the _____.

TOPIC 5: Skin Elasticity

1. Skin elasticity can be traced to protein fibers called _____ and _____ within the _____.

2. _____ fibers give support to structures found in the dermis.

3. _____ gives the skin its elasticity, flexibility, and the ability to regain its shape after stretching.

4. Healthy skin will regain its former shape almost immediately after _____.

5. One of the most outstanding characteristics of aged skin is its loss of _____.

TOPIC 6: Skin Color

1. The color of the skin depends on the _____ supply and _____.

2. _____ is the primary source of skin color; the pigment grains are deposited in the _____ of the epidermis and the _____ layer of the dermis.

3. Special cells called _____ produce the pigment granules scattered throughout the skin layers. These granules are called _____ and produce the complex protein melanin.

4. Melanin is a _____ pigment that serves as the skin's protective screen from the sun's rays.

5. The color of pigment is a _____ trait that varies among races and nationalities and varies from person to person.

6. _____ skin contains more melanin than _____ skin.

TOPIC 7: Glands of the Skin

The skin contains two types of duct glands that extract material from the blood to form new substances.

1. The _____ or _____ glands consist of a coiled base and a tube-like duct that ends at the skin surface and forms the _____ . The parts of the body that have the most numerous supply of these glands are the palms, soles, _____ , and _____ .

2. The sweat glands help to regulate _____ and to eliminate _____ from the body.

3. The excretion of sweat is under the control of the _____ system.

4. Sweat gland activity is increased by _____ , _____ , _____ , and certain _____ .

5. The average daily elimination of salt-containing liquid by the sweat pores is _____ to _____ pints.

6. The _____ or _____ glands are connected to the _____ . These glands consist of little sacs with _____ that open into the hair follicle, where they secrete _____ .

7. _____ is a semi-fluid, oily substance produced by the oil glands that lubricates the skin and preserves the softness of the hair.

8. The primary function of sebum is to _____ _____ .

9. When sebum hardens and blocks the duct, a _____ is formed.

10. Oil glands are found on all parts of the body except the _____ and _____ .

TOPIC 8: Absorption of the Skin

1. The skin serves as a protective barrier to _____ and chemical absorption.

2. _____ absorption occurs through the skin cells, hair follicles, sebaceous glands, and sudoriferous glands.

3. The pockets in the skin created by hair follicles and pores allow the entry of certain _____ and _____ into the body. Two examples are _____ and skin _____ .

67

TOPIC 9: Functions of the Skin

1. The principal functions of the skin are _____, sensation, _____, excretion, secretion, and absorption.

2. Match the following descriptions with the correct skin function.

   _____ sebum lubricates the skin and hair   a) sensation

   _____ protects the body from environment changes   b) heat regulation

   _____ water is lost by perspiration   c) absorption

   _____ helps the body avoid injury and bacteria   d) protection

   _____ facilitates acceptance of hormonal and lanolin creams   e) excretion

   _____ sends messages and stimulates a response   f) secretion

TOPIC 10: Disorders of the Skin

Barbers are not licensed to perform treatments for medical reasons; however, they *are* permitted to perform prevention and maintenance treatments for certain skin conditions.

1. Three skin conditions that barbers may treat through facial services are _____ skin, _____ skin, and minor _____ conditions.

2. Barbers need to be able to recognize _____ such as moles and warts, or skin conditions that may be aggravated by facial or shaving procedures.

3. Some skin and scalp disorders may be treated in cooperation with or under the supervision of a physician or _____.

4. _____ are signs or indications of disease.

5. Symptoms of skin disorders are generally divided into two groups: _____ symptoms and _____ symptoms.

6. Subjective symptoms are symptoms that can be felt, such as _____, _____, or _____.

7. Objective symptoms are those that can be observed by anyone, such as _____ or _____.

TOPIC 11: Lesions of the Skin

1. Lesions such as _____, _____, or _____ are symptoms that barbers see in the performance of their work. It is important for barbers to be able to differentiate between common or _____ skin conditions and serious or _____ disorders.

2. A _____ is a structural change in the tissues caused by injury or disease. Barbers are concerned with only _____ and _____ lesions.

3. _____ lesions are characterized by flat, non-palpable changes in skin color, elevations formed by fluid in a cavity, or elevated, palpable solid masses.

68

4. Review the following illustrations, then study the examples and label the name of each primary lesion.

Terms: Bulla, Macule, Papule, Pustule, Tubercle, Tumor, Vesicle, Wheal

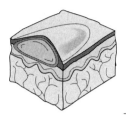

_____

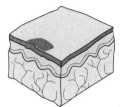

_____

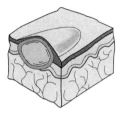

_____

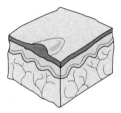

_____

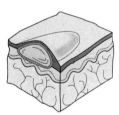

_____

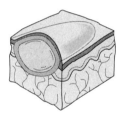

_____

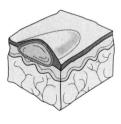

_____

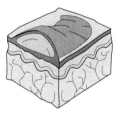

_____

5. Review the following lesion descriptions, then match each to the correct name from the list.

_____ a large blister containing a watery fluid

_____ sac containing fluid or semi-fluid substance, above or below the skin

_____ small, discolored spot or patch on the skin surface

_____ small, elevated pimple with no fluid, but may develop pus

_____ an inflamed pimple containing pus

_____ abnormal, solid lump that projects above or lies within the skin

_____ abnormal cell mass resulting from excessive cell multiplication

_____ small blister or sac containing clear fluid

_____ itchy, swollen lesion lasting only a few hours

a) macule

b) vesicle

c) bulla

d) tubercule

e) wheal

f) tumor

g) cyst

h) papule

i) pustule

6. Secondary lesions are characterized by a collection of material on the skin. Examples of secondary lesions are _____ , _____ , _____ , _____ , and _____ .

7. Review the following illustrations, study the examples, and label the name of each secondary lesion.

    Terms: crust, excoriation, fissure, scale, scar, ulcer

_____   _____   _____

_____   _____   _____

8. Review the following secondary lesion descriptions, then select the correct name from the list. Choices may be used more than once.

_____ chapped hands or lips	a) scar
_____ technical term is cicatrix	b) crust
_____ accumulation of dry or greasy flakes	c) excoriation
_____ thick scar resulting from excessive fibrous tissue growth	d) fissure
_____ accumulation of dead cells that forms over a wound	e) keloid
_____ crack in the skin that penetrates to the dermis	f) scale
_____ skin sore caused by scratching or scraping	
_____ raised mark that forms after an injury	
_____ also known as a scab	

9. A hypertrophy is an abnormal growth of skin tissue that is usually _____ or harmless.

10. A _____ is a superficial, thickened patch of skin caused by continued pressure or friction and is also known as a _____.

11. A small, brownish spot on the skin ranging in color from pale tan to brown or black is called a _____.

12. If a mole grows in size, gets darker, or becomes sore or scaly, _____ is needed.

13. Barbers should not treat or remove _____ from _____.

14. A _____ is caused by a virus. It is the technical term for _____ and is infectious to the person who has one and can spread from one location to another.

TOPIC 12: Pigmentations of the Skin

1. The _____ of the skin may be affected by internal factors within the body or from external conditions such as prolonged sun exposure.

2. Liver spots, or _____, are caused by increased deposits of pigment in the skin.

3. _____ is the technical term for freckles.

4. A skin disorder characterized by abnormal white patches caused by a burn or congenital pigmentation defects is called _____. Two types of this disorder are _____ and _____.

5. A _____ is a small or large malformation of the skin due to abnormal pigmentation or dilated capillaries. It is commonly known as a _____.

6. An abnormal brown or wine-colored skin discoloration with a generally circular and irregular shape is called a _____.

7. A change in the pigmentation of the skin caused by exposure to the sun or ultraviolet rays is called a _____ .

TOPIC 13: Skin Inflammations

Dermatitis is the general term for an inflammatory condition of the skin.

1. _____ is an inflammatory skin disease that may be acute or chronic and present in the form of _____ or _____ lesions. This skin inflammation is frequently accompanied by _____ or _____ and should be referred to a physician for treatment. Its cause is _____ .

2. A recurring viral infection that produces fever blisters or cold sores around the lips or nostrils is known as _____ . The blisters rarely last more than a _____ , but the condition is _____ .

3. _____ is a chronic, inflammatory skin disease that is characterized by dry _____ patches covered with coarse _____ . It is _____ contagious and the cause is _____ .

4. An inflammatory skin disease, characterized by a small, red papule followed by the formation of a pustule, vesicle, and hard swelling, is an indication of _____ . It is accompanied by _____ and _____ and is _____ . One way in which it can be spread in the barbershop is through the use of an _____ shaving brush.

5. _____ is a skin inflammation caused by exposure to poison ivy, poison oak, or poison sumac leaves. It can be spread from one person to another by _____ contact.

6. _____ is an eruptive skin infection that is caused by contact with chemicals or tints. This is an _____ disorder or disease that may be minimized by using rubber gloves or protective creams.

TOPIC 14: Disorders of the Sebaceous Glands

Barbers should be able to identify common disorders of the sebaceous glands.

1. _____ is a skin disorder characterized by chronic inflammation of the sebaceous glands from retained secretions.

2. The two basic types of acne are acne _____ and acne _____ .

3. Which type of acne refers to common pimples? _____

4. The cause of acne is generally held to be _____ in nature.

5. Dry, scaly skin caused by the absolute or partial deficiency of sebum is called _____ .

6. A mass of hardened sebum and dead cells in a hair follicle that creates a blockage is called a _____ .

7. _____ comedones, also known as _____, occur when excess oil in the follicles is exposed to oxygen.

8. _____ comedones, also known as _____, do not have a follicular opening for oxygen exposure.

9. _____, also known as milk spots, are small, benign, whitish bumps that occur when dead skin is trapped in the surface of the skin.

10. A _____ is a sebaceous cyst or fatty tumor filled with sebum. It is a _____ tumor of the sebaceous glands and is sometimes called a _____.

11. _____ is a chronic inflammatory congestion of the cheeks and nose. Its cause is _____, but factors such as hot liquids, spicy foods, alcohol, extreme temperatures, or _____ are known to aggravate the condition in some individuals.

12. Seborrhea is a skin condition due to _____ and excessive _____ of the _____ glands. Itching, burning, and an oily or shiny nose, forehead, or scalp indicates its presence.

TOPIC 15: Disorders of the Sudoriferous Glands

1. _____ refers to foul-smelling perspiration.

2. _____ refers to a lack of perspiration.

3. _____ is excessive perspiration.

4. _____ is the technical term for prickly heat.

TOPIC 16: Skin Cancer

Skin cancer from overexposure to the sun comes in three forms that vary in severity.

1. _____ cell carcinoma is the most common and the least severe type of skin cancer and is often characterized by light or pearly _____.

2. _____ cell carcinoma is more serious than basal cell carcinoma and is often characterized by scaly _____ or nodules.

3. _____ is the _____ common but most serious form of skin cancer. It is characterized by dark brown or _____ patches on the skin that may appear jagged, raised, or uneven in texture.

4. Barbers should not attempt to diagnosis skin disorders, but they should be aware of _____ in their clients' _____ so they can tactfully suggest that the client seeks the advice of a dermatologist.

5. When checking or observing existing lesions or hypertrophies, look for changes in any of the following: A, _____; B, _____; C, _____; D, _____; E, _____.

TOPIC 17: Health of the Skin

1. _____ is the major factor involved in maintaining the skin's overall health and appearance.

2. Proper and beneficial dietary choices help to regulate _____, _____ production, and the _____ of cells.

3. Water helps to sustain the health of the _____, aids in the elimination of toxins and waste, helps to _____ the body's temperature, and aids in proper digestion.

Chapter 11: Properties and Disorders of the Hair and Scalp

Word Review

alopecia	hair density	lanugo
amino acids	hair elasticity	melanin
cortex	hair porosity	salt bonds
cowlick	hair root	sebaceous glands
cuticle	hair shaft	trichology
follicle	hair texture	vellus
folliculitis	hydrogen bonds	wave pattern
hair bulb	keratin	whorl

TOPIC 1: Introduction

A technical understanding of the structure of hair is vitally important to barbers so that they will be able to provide knowledgeable and professional service to clients. Knowledge and analysis of the client's hair, tactful suggestions for its improvement, and a sincere interest in maintaining its health and appearance should be the concern of every barber and stylist.

1. The scientific study of hair, its disorders, and its care is called _____.

2. In addition to being a form of adornment, hair protects the head from _____, _____, and _____.

TOPIC 2: Hair Structure

1. Hair is an _____ of the skin in the form of a slender, thread-like outgrowth of the skin and scalp.

2. Hair is composed chiefly of a protein called _____.

3. Full-grown human hair is divided into two parts: the hair _____ and the hair _____.

4. The hair _____ is that portion of the hair found beneath the skin surface and enclosed within the _____.

5. The hair _____ is that portion of the hair that extends above the skin surface.

6. The main structures of the hair root are the follicle, bulb, dermal papilla, arrector pili muscle, and sebaceous glands. Using these identifiers, label the following illustration.

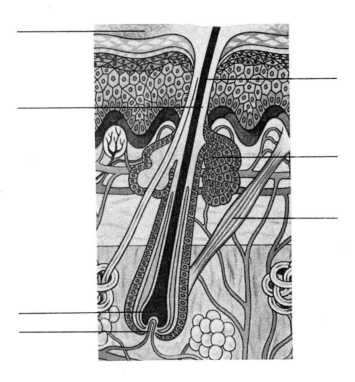

7. Review the following characteristics of the structures of the hair, then match the characteristics to the correct word or term. Choices may be used more than once.

_____ thickened, club-like structure

_____ set at an angle

_____ sac-like structure with ducts

_____ cone-shaped elevation

_____ involuntary muscle fiber

_____ forms the lower part of the hair root

_____ secretes sebum

_____ fits into the hair bulb

_____ depression or pocket in the skin or scalp

_____ vital to regeneration of the hair

_____ fits over the papilla

_____ encases the hair root

_____ attached to the underside and base of the follicle

a) follicle

b) bulb

c) dermal papilla

d) arrector pili

e) sebaceous gland

8. As long as the _____ is healthy and well nourished, new hair will grow.

9. The production of sebum may be influenced by _____,
   _____, the condition of the _____, and
   _____.

10. The structures of the hair shaft are the cortex, cuticle, and medulla. Using these identifiers, label the following illustration.

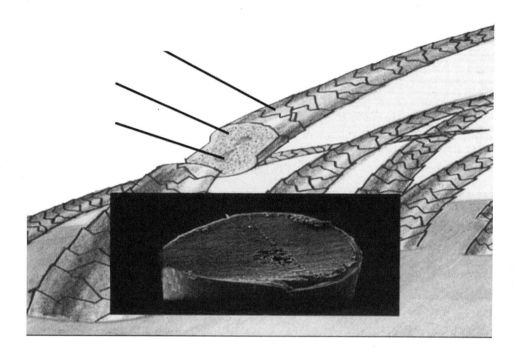

11. The outermost layer of the hair is the _____, which consists of an overlapping layer of transparent, scale-like cells that point away from the _____ toward the hair _____.

12. A healthy, compact _____ layer is the hair's primary defense against _____.

13. Certain chemical solutions soften and raise the cuticle scales to allow for _____ into the cortex.

14. Chemicals with an _____ pH can penetrate the cuticle layer.

15. The _____ is the middle layer of the hair and is a fibrous _____ core.

16. The cortex contains _____ pigment and provides _____, _____, and natural color to the hair.

17. The changes that take place in the hair during chemical services occur within the _____.

18. The innermost layer of the hair shaft is the _____.

19. Hair that is very fine or naturally blond may not have a _____.

20. In most cases, mature male _____ hair contains a medulla.

TOPIC 3: Hair Protein

Hair is composed of protein that grows from cells that originate within the hair follicle. This is where the hair shaft begins.

1. As the newly formed cells mature, they fill up with a fibrous protein called _____.

2. As the cells begin the journey upward through the follicle, they mature through a process called _____.

3. When the hair shaft emerges from the scalp, the cells are completely _____ and no longer living.

4. Hair is approximately _____ percent protein.

5. Protein is made up of long chains of amino acids, which are made up of _____.

6. The elements found in human hair are _____, _____, _____, _____, and _____. These five elements are referred to as the _____ elements, and the chemical composition of average hair is _____ percent carbon, _____ percent oxygen, _____ percent hydrogen, _____ percent nitrogen, and _____ percent sulfur.

7. Light hair contains _____ carbon and hydrogen and _____ oxygen and sulfur; dark hair has _____ carbon and _____ oxygen and sulfur.

Hair is a complex structure that varies from one person to another; however, all hair types have certain common factors that include proteins, amino acids, polypeptide chains, and bonds.

1. _____ are organic compounds necessary for life that are made of long chains of chemical units known as _____.

2. Each amino acid is joined _____ in a definite order by chemical bonds known as _____ or _____ bonds.

3. The peptide bonds are the strongest _____ bonds in the cortex as they join each amino acid to form the polypeptide chain; most of the _____ and _____ of the hair is attributed to these chemical bonds.

4. Peptide bonds can be broken through over-stretching or strong _____ or _____ solutions.

5. Once end bonds are broken, there is no way of _____ them.

6. A long chain of amino acids joined by peptide bonds is called a _____ or _____.

7. Polypeptide chains intertwine to create a coil or spiral of protein called a _____.

8. Polypeptide chains are cross-linked by three types of _____ or _____ bonds to form a ladder-like structure.

9. Side bonds, also known as _____ consist of hydrogen, salt, and disulfide bonds; these bonds account for the strength and elasticity of human hair.

10. _____ bonds are physical side bonds that are easily broken by _____ or _____; they are also known as _____ bonds or _____. Water, dilute _____, neutral, and _____ solutions will break hydrogen bonds; _____ and _____ acids will reform them.

11. A _____ bond is also a physical ionic bond and will react to changes in _____. Salt bonds are easily broken by strong _____ or _____ solutions.

12. _____ bonds are covalent bonds that are also known as _____ bonds, _____ bonds, or _____.

13. Disulfide bonds are stronger than hydrogen or salt bonds and account for one-_____ of the hair's total strength.

14. Disulfide bonds create _____ side bonds between the polypeptide chains; therefore, _____ solutions are required to change or restructure them.

15. Chemicals such as _____ thioglycolate and _____ hydroxide will break disulfide bonds.

TOPIC 4: Hair Pigment

Natural hair color is the result of the melanin pigment found within the cortex.

1. The two types of melanin are _____ and _____.

2. Eumelanin provides _____ and _____ color to hair.

3. _____ provides natural hair colors that range from _____ and ginger to yellow and light blonde tones.

4. All natural color is dependent on the _____ of eumelanin to pheomelanin and the _____ and _____ of the pigment granules.

5. The number of hairs on the head varies with the color of the hair. Match the following hair colors with their average number of hairs.

_____ blond   a) 80,000

_____ brown   b) 108,000

_____ black   c) 110,000

_____ red   d) 140,000

TOPIC 5: Wave Pattern

1. The wave pattern of the hair refers to the amount of _____ in the hair strand.

2. Wave pattern is described as _____, _____, _____, or extremely _____.

3. Each of the four wave patterns can be found in each _____ or _____ group.

4. There are three general shapes of hair. Although wavy, straight, or curly hair has been found in all shapes, a cross-sectional view of hair reveals that straight hair is usually _____, wavy hair is usually _____, and extremely curly hair is usually almost _____.

TOPIC 6: Hair Growth

The three main types of hair on the body are vellus or lanugo hair, primary terminal hair, and secondary terminal hair.

1. The short, fine hair found on the cheeks, forehead, and most of the body that helps in the evaporation of perspiration is called _____ or _____ hair.

2. _____ terminal hair is the short, thick hair that grows on the eyebrows and eyelashes.

3. The long hair found on the scalp, beard, chest, back, and legs is called _____ terminal hair.

4. The average rate of growth of healthy hair on the scalp is about _____" per month.

5. Hair _____ is not increased by shaving, trimming, cutting, singeing, or by applying ointments or oils.

6. _____ act as lubricants to the hair shaft but do not feed the hair.

7. It is normal to lose an average of _____ to _____ scalp hairs per day; eyebrow hairs and eyelashes are replaced every four to five _____.

It is important when cutting and styling hair to consider the hair's natural growth patterns.

8. A _____ is hair that flows in the same direction as a result of the follicles being arranged and sloping in a uniform manner. When two such streams slope in opposite directions, they form a natural _____ in the hair.

9. A _____ is hair that forms in a _____ or swirl pattern, most often at the _____.

10. A _____ is a tuft of hair that stands straight up.

In normal and healthy hair, each individual strand goes through a cycle of events: growth, fall, and replacement.

11. The three phases of the hair growth cycle are the _____, _____, and _____ phases.

12. Review the following characteristics of the hair growth cycle, then identify the characteristic as being representative of the anagen, catagen, or telogen phase. Choices may be used more than once.

_____ phase that is a transition period

_____ the growth phase

_____ new hair is produced

_____ accounts for 1 percent of scalp hair

_____ the resting phase

_____ stem cells manufacture new keratinized cells

_____ final phase of the hair cycle

_____ accounts for about 10 percent of scalp hair

_____ lasts one to three weeks

_____ accounts for about 90 percent of scalp hair

_____ the hair bulb disappears

_____ lasts from three to five years

_____ the shrunken root end forms a rounded club

_____ follicle makes new germ cells

_____ lasts from three to six months

13. To describe the manner in which new hair replaces old hair, number the following in the order in which they occur.

_____ The bulb moves upward in the follicle.

_____ The bulb loosens and separates from the papilla.

_____ The hair moves slowly to the surface, where it is shed.

_____ The new hair is formed from a growing point at the root around the papilla.

TOPIC 7: Hair Analysis

Barbering services include a variety of applications that benefit from a barber's ability to analyze the condition of their client's hair.

1. Barbers should be able to analyze the hair's _____, _____, _____, and _____.

2. Hair analysis requires _____ and _____.

3. The senses used to analyze the hair are sight, _____, hearing, and smell.

4. The degree of coarseness or fineness of individual hair strands relates to hair _____ and is measured by the _____ of the hair strand.

5. Hair texture is classified as _____, _____, or _____.

6. _____ hair has the largest diameter, _____ hair is considered normal, and _____ hair has the smallest diameter.

7. _____ hair, whether coarse, medium, or fine, has a hard, _____ finish because the cuticle scales lie flat against the hair shaft; _____ processing usually takes longer for this hair texture.

8. Describe one method to determine hair texture using the sense of touch. _____ _____

9. Hair _____ measures the number of individual hair strands per square inch of scalp area.

10. The density of the hair is classified as _____, _____, or _____ or as high, medium, and low density.

11. The average hair density is approximately _____ per square inch, with the average head of hair containing about _____ individual strands.

12. Hair _____ is the ability of the hair to absorb moisture.

13. The degree of porosity is directly related to the condition of the _____ layer of the hair.

14. A compact cuticle layer is more _____ to penetration; porous hair has a _____ cuticle layer that easily absorbs water.

15. Porosity levels of hair are classified as _____, _____, and _____ or as average, low, and high porosity.

16. Moderate or average porosity is considered _____.

17. _____ hair has a high or porous porosity level.

18. _____ hair has a poor or low porosity level.

19. How can the porosity level of the hair be determined? _____ _____

20. How does resistant hair feel? _____

21. What does porous hair feel like? _____

22. What are some indications of an over-porous hair condition? _____ _____

23. Hair _____ is the ability of the hair to stretch and return to its original length without breaking.

24. _____ hair with normal elasticity may stretch up to 50 percent of its original length and return to that length without breaking.

25. Hair elasticity is an indication of the strength of the _____ in the hair.

26. Hair with _____ elasticity is brittle and breaks easily.

27. How is a hair elasticity test performed? _____
_____

TOPIC 8: Hair Loss

Over 63 million people in the United States suffer from abnormal hair loss.

1. _____ is the technical term for any abnormal hair loss.

2. Four primary forms of alopecia are _____ alopecia, alopecia _____, alopecia _____, and alopecia _____.

3. Review the following characteristics of certain forms of alopecia, and match the descriptions with the most correct form.

    _____ also known as male pattern baldness

    _____ normal loss of scalp hair occurring in old age

    _____ sudden falling out of hair in round patches

    _____ total scalp hair loss

    _____ may be the result of a nervous condition

    _____ occurs as a result of genetics

    _____ complete loss of body hair

    _____ hair loss during the teen years

    _____ hair loss caused by syphilis

    _____ may be an autoimmune disease

    _____ may be the result of hormonal changes

    _____ converts terminal hair to vellus hair

    _____ may or may not be permanent hair loss

    a) androgenic alopecia

    b) alopecia prematura

    c) alopecia totalis

    d) alopecia senilis

    e) alopecia syphilitica

    f) alopecia areata

    g) alopecia universalis

4. Two hair loss treatments that have been proven to stimulate hair growth and that are approved by the FDA are _____ and _____.

5. _____ is an oral prescription medication for men only.

6. Transplants, or _____, are one of the most common permanent hair replacement techniques.

7. Only licensed _____ may perform transplants or hair grafting.

8. Barbers can offer non-medical or non-surgical options to their clients such as wigs, hair _____ systems, and hair _____ or _____.

TOPIC 9: Scalp Disorders

1. Common disorders of the scalp include _____ , _____ parasitic infections, _____ parasitic infestations, and _____ infections.

2. The technical term for the presence of small, white scales on the scalp and hair is _____; the common term is _____.

3. The two principal types of dandruff are pityriasis _____ and pityriasis _____.

4. Classic dandruff is characterized by scalp irritation, large flakes, and an itchy scalp; it is known as pityriasis _____.

5. Dry dandruff may be the result of poor _____, lack of _____ stimulation, emotional and glandular disturbances, improper diet, and poor personal hygiene.

6. Treatments for classic dandruff may include the use of mild or medicated shampoos, _____ and treatments, and _____ or medicated scalp ointments.

7. _____ is characterized by an accumulation of greasy or waxy scales mixed with sebum irritation; if torn off, _____ or _____ secretion may follow. _____ is advisable for clients with this condition.

8. The latest research has determined that dandruff _____ contagious.

9. The medical term for ringworm is _____.

10. Ringworm is caused by _____ organisms; it is characterized by itching, scales, and _____ lesions that heal first in the _____.

11. All forms of tinea are _____ and all cases should be referred to a _____.

12. _____ is commonly known as ringworm of the scalp.

13. Tinea sycosis, also known as _____, is a fungal infection occurring over the _____ area of the face; in severe cases, _____ form around the hair _____ and rupture, forming crusts.

14. Tinea _____, also known as tinea _____ or _____ ringworm, is characterized by dry, yellowish crusts on the scalp with a musty odor.

15. The two most common animal parasitic infestations that barbers see in the barbershop are _____ and _____.

16. Pediculosis capitis is the infestation of the hair and scalp with _____ .

17. Pediculosis capitis is transmitted from one person to another by contact with infested hats, _____ , _____ , and other personal items.

18. Cases of head lice _____ be treated in the barbershop.

19. _____ is a highly contagious skin disease caused by the _____ that is characterized by itching, vesicles, and pustules.

20. Staphylococcal infections that barbers may encounter in the barbershop are _____ , _____ , and _____ .

21. A chronic bacterial infection involving the follicles of the beard and mustache areas is called _____ .

22. Sycosis vulgaris is transmitted through unsanitary _____ or _____ and is characterized by _____ and _____ pierced by hairs; this requires _____ treatment.

23. A _____ or boil is an acute _____ infection of a _____ that produces constant pain.

24. A _____ is a deep-seated bacterial infection in the _____ tissue that is larger than a furuncle.

25. Clients with a furuncle or a carbuncle should be referred to a _____ .

26. _____ and _____ barbae are inflammations of the _____ caused by bacterial or viral infection, ingrown hair, or _____ .

27. Staphylococcus aureus and yeast are common bacterial causes of _____ .

28. Mechanical irritation caused by improper _____ combined with bacteria can also cause folliculitis.

29. Pseudofolliculitis barbae is also known as _____ and resembles folliculitis without the _____ .

30. _____ is prevented by shaving in the direction of the _____ and by avoiding _____ shaving.

TOPIC 10: Hair Disorders

1. Hair disorders are usually _____ conditions.

2. Review the following hair disorders, then match each with the correct technical term from the list.

_____ technical term for gray hair

_____ exists at or before birth

_____ alternating bands of gray and pigmented hair

_____ abnormal growth of terminal hair

_____ due to the natural aging process and genetics

_____ knotted hair

_____ term for split ends

_____ term for beaded hair

_____ brittle hair

a) hypertrichosis

b) trichoptilosis

c) trichorrhexis nodosa

d) canities

e) monilethrix

f) acquired canities

g) congenital canities

h) fragilitas crinium

i) ringed hair

Chapter 12: Treatment of the Hair and Scalp

Word Review

conditioner   liquid dry shampoo   shampoo
draping   medicated shampoo   tonics
dry or powder shampoo   scalp conditioner
hair conditioners   scalp steam

TOPIC 1: Introduction

1. The treatment of the hair and scalp includes regular _____, scalp massage services, and special treatments for _____ and _____ conditions.

2. These services help to ensure the _____ of the client's hair and scalp from one shop visit to another.

3. The purpose of a shampoo product and service is to _____ the scalp and hair.

4. Shampoo products are specially formulated solutions for the hair and scalp that _____ contain the harsh alkalis found in soaps and detergents.

5. Conditioners *refers to either* _____ conditioners or _____ conditioners.

TOPIC 2: Draping

1. The comfort and _____ of the client must always be considered during barbering services.

2. The two main types of drapes used to perform barbering services are the _____ or plastic cape, also known as _____ cape, and the haircutting cape, also known as a _____.

3. Waterproof capes are used to protect the client's skin and clothing from liquids during _____ and _____ processes.

4. The preferred haircutting capes are made of nylon or synthetic materials because these are more effective in shedding _____ and _____ hair.

5. The method of draping to be used depends on the _____ being provided.

6. List the important steps for draping a client for any type of service.

    1. _____

    2. _____

3. _____

4. _____

5. _____

7. The purpose of the towel or neck strip is to _____
_____ and to _____ .

8. The application of a barrier between the client's skin and the drape is a requirement of _____
_____ .

9. Wet hair services include shampooing, _____ , and all chemical
applications.

10. Fill in the blanks to list the steps use to drape a client for a wet hair service.

   1. Fold a towel in a lengthwise and _____ manner. Place the towel lengthwise
   across the client's shoulders, _____ beneath the chin.

   2. Drape a plastic or waterproof cape over the towel and fasten it at the back so that the cape
   does not touch the client's skin. Position and _____ the top edge of the towel
   down over the neckline of the cape.

   3. Optional: Place another towel _____ the cape and secure it in front with a
   chair cloth clip.

Haircut draping requires a towel or neck strip and a nylon or synthetic cape.

11. Fill in the blanks to list the steps used in draping a client for a haircut service.

   1. Drape the cape loosely across the client's chest and shoulders. Place the _____
   around the client's neck from _____ to _____ . Hold one end
   of the neckstrip against the client's skin at the back or side of the neck while wrapping the rest of
   the strip. Secure the second neckstrip end by tucking it neatly into the rest of the neckstrip.

   2. Lift the _____ or cape from across the client's shoulders, slide it into place
   around the neck, and fasten at the back of the neck.

   3. Fold and flatten the top edge of the neckstrip over the _____ of the cape to
   prevent the client's skin from touching the drape.

TOPIC 3: The Shampoo Service

1. The shampoo service requires proper draping and _____ of the client, proper
_____ in the shampoo procedure, and proper body positioning of the barber.

2. The two methods used for shampooing and rinsing are the _____ method and
_____ method.

3. The _____ method requires the client to bend his head forward over the
shampoo bowl.

88

4. Good posture at the shampoo sink helps to prevent muscle aches, back strain, and fatigue. List four suggestions to help maintain a good posture while shampooing.

   1. _____

   _____

   2. _____

   _____

   3. _____

   _____

   4. _____

   _____

5. Fill in the blanks to complete the list of reasons why a client may find fault with the shampoo service.

   a) improper _____ selection

   b) _____ scalp massage

   c) _____ water temperatures, either too hot or too cold

   d) shampoo or water that runs onto _____ face, ears, or eyes

   e) _____ or soiling the client's clothing

   f) scraping or scratching the client's scalp with _____

   g) improper hair _____

   h) insufficient cleansing and _____

TOPIC 4: Product Selection

It is essential that the barber be knowledgeable about the products used in the shop. Always read product labels and follow the manufacturer's directions. To determine which product to use, perform a hair and scalp analysis.

1. Characteristics of the hair and scalp that should be considered before choosing products are:

   a) condition of the _____: dry, oily, normal, abrasions, or disorders present.

   b) condition of the _____: dry, brittle, fragile, oily, normal, or chemically treated.

   c) hair density: _____, _____, or _____.

   d) hair texture: _____, _____, or _____.

   e) hair porosity: _____, _____, or _____.

   f) hair elasticity: _____, _____, or _____.

2. Practice and experience help barbering students to learn the effects of certain products on the hair and scalp. For example, moisturizing shampoos are not _____ enough to cleanse an oily scalp and hair condition.

3. Water used in a shampoo service should be comfortably _____ for the client.

4. Following a warm water rinse to dampen the hair, the shampoo product should be dispensed into the barber's hand and then _____

_____ .

5. All shampoo movements must be executed with the _____ of the fingers.

6. List the steps of the proper way to massage the scalp during a shampoo.

   1. _____

   _____

   2. _____

   _____

   3. _____

   _____

   4. _____

   _____

   5. _____

   _____

7. Fill in the blanks where necessary to complete the steps used in the shampoo service.

   1. Seat the client in a comfortable and relaxed position.

   2. Drape the client according to the textbook or instructor's procedures.

   3. _____ with the client about products, hair and scalp problems, or any questions they have about their hair or scalp.

   4. _____ the condition of the client's hair and scalp. Briefly _____ the scalp to loosen epidermal scales, debris, and scalp tissues.

   5. Decide on the type of products to be used.

   6. Position the client for the shampoo service. Drape the back of the cape _____ .

   7. Wet the hair with _____ water.

   8. Apply shampoo to all areas of the scalp.

   9. Massage the scalp for several minutes.

   10. Rinse the hair _____ with warm water and repeat second lathering and rinsing if necessary.

   11. _____ the hair.

   12. Raise client to a sitting position and lightly _____ the hair; wipe client's face and _____ if necessary.

   14. Comb hair into position for cutting.

90

8. Fill in the blanks where necessary to complete the steps used for a liquid dry shampoo procedure.

    1. _____ the hair thoroughly and comb it lightly.

    2. Part the hair into small _____.

    3. Saturate a piece of cotton with the liquid dry shampoo, squeeze it out lightly, and apply it to the _____ along each part line. Follow by swiftly _____ the scalp with a towel along the same area.

    4. Saturate more cotton with the product and apply down the length of the hair _____.

    5. Rub the hair strands with a towel to remove the soil.

    6. Re-moisten the hair lightly with liquid and comb it into the desired style.

9. Explain the procedure used to perform a powder dry shampoo. _____

_____

_____.

TOPIC 5: Scalp and Hair Treatments

The purpose of scalp and hair treatments is to preserve the health and appearance of the hair and scalp. Scalp treatments may be given separately or combined with hair treatments.

1. Depending on the client's needs, the scalp treatment may include cleansing with a suitable shampoo; massage with the hands or _____; use of other electrical appliances; or the application of _____ preparations, such as hair tonics, astringents, _____, or ointments.

2. Do not suggest a scalp treatment if _____ or _____ are present.

3. A _____ prepares the scalp for massage manipulations and treatments.

4. Steam _____ the pores, _____ the scalp and hair, and increases _____.

5. If a scalp steamer is not available, _____ can be used.

6. Explain how to prepare a steam towel. _____

_____

_____.

7. The massage techniques used to perform scalp treatments are more thorough than those used in the _____ service.

8. List the benefits of a thorough scalp massage.

    a) _____

    b) _____

    c) _____

d) _____

e) _____

9. When performing scalp massage, firm pressure is applied on the _____ strokes.

10. Firm _____ movements loosen the scalp tissues and help to improve the health of hair and scalp by _____ the blood's circulation to the scalp and hair papillae.

11. Massage manipulations should be _____ and _____.

12. The length of the fingers, the balls of the fingertips, and the cushions of the palms all help to stimulate _____, _____, and _____ in the scalp area.

13. Fill in the blanks to complete the steps and actions involved in the scalp massage procedure.

1. Place the fingertips of each hand at the hairline on each side of the client's head, hands pointing upward. Firmly slide the fingers _____, spreading the fingertips. Continue until the fingers meet at the center or _____ of the scalp. Repeat three or four times.

2. Place the fingers of each hand on the sides of the head, behind the ears. Use a _____ movement of the thumbs to massage from behind the ears toward the crown. Repeat four or five times. Move the fingers until both thumbs meet at the _____ at the back of neck. Rotate the thumbs upward toward the crown.

3. Move to the _____ of the client. Place the left hand at the back of the head. Place the thumb and fingers of the right hand against and over the forehead, just above the eyebrows. With the cushion tips of the thumb and fingers of the right hand, use a _____ movement to massage slowly and _____ across the top of the head toward the crown while keeping the left hand in a fixed position at the back of the head. Repeat four or five times.

4. Move _____ the client. Place the hands on each side of the head at the _____ hairline. Rotate the fingertips three times. On the fourth rotation, apply a quick, upward twist, firm enough to _____ the scalp. Continue this movement on the sides and top of the scalp. Repeat three or four times.

5. Place the fingers of each hand _____ of each ear. Rotate the fingers upward from behind the ears to the crown. Repeat three or four times. Move the fingers toward the back of the head and repeat the movement with both hands. Apply rotary movements in a/an _____ direction toward the crown.

6. Place one hand at either side of the head. Keep the fingers close together and position at the hairline above the ears. Firmly move the hands directly upward to the _____ of the head in a _____ movement. Repeat four times. Move the hands to _____ above the ears and repeat the movement. Move the hands to the back of the ears.

14. Review Table 12-2 in the textbook to fill in the blanks in the following table.

MASSAGE AND ITS INFLUENCE ON THE SCALP

Massage Movements	Muscles	Nerves	Arteries
_____	auricularis superior	posterior auricular	_____ _____
_____	auricularis osterior	_____ _____	occipital
_____ _____	frontalis	supra-orbital	frontal
_____	_____	supra-orbital	frontal and parietal
_____	auricularis posterior	_____ _____	posterior auricular and Parietal
_____ _____	_____ _____ _____	temporal auricular	frontal and parietal

15. A/An _____ is an electrical tool used to perform a stimulating scalp massage through the cushions of the fingertips.

16. When using a vibrator on the scalp, the _____ of the vibrations, the duration of the vibrations, and the _____ need to be regulated.

17. The purpose of a general scalp treatment is to keep the scalp and hair clean and healthy. Fill in the blanks where necessary to complete the steps for a general scalp treatment for normal hair and scalp.

    1. Drape the client.

    2. Brush the hair for a few minutes to _____.

    3. Part the hair and apply a scalp _____ or ointment directly to the scalp with a cotton pledget.

    4. Apply _____ lamp for 3 to 5 minutes.

    5. Massage the scalp for _____ minutes.

6. Shampoo the hair and towel dry.

7. Optional step: Stimulate the scalp with high-frequency current for 2 to 3 minutes.

8. Apply a suitable _____ lotion or tonic and work it well into the scalp.

9. Comb and style the hair.

18. Inactivity of the oil glands or the excessive removal of natural oil produces dry hair and scalp conditions. Fill in the blanks where necessary to complete the steps for a dry hair and scalp treatment.

1. Drape the client.

2. Brush the client's hair.

3. Massage and _____ the scalp for 3 to 5 minutes.

4. Apply a _____ preparation for this condition.

5. _____ the scalp with hot towels or steamer for 7 to 10 minutes.

6. Shampoo the hair with a _____ shampoo suitable for dry scalp and hair.

7. Towel-dry the hair, making sure the _____ is thoroughly _____.

8. Apply scalp cream _____ with a rotary, frictional motion.

9. Apply an infrared lamp over the scalp for _____ minutes.

10. Stimulate the scalp with _____ high-frequency current using a glass rake electrode for about 5 minutes.

11. Rinse the hair thoroughly.

12. Comb the hair into the desired style.

19. Never use a scalp or hair treatment product that contains _____ before applying high-frequency current; such products can only be safely applied _____ the high-frequency treatment.

20 The main cause of an oily scalp is overactive sebaceous glands. The type of scalp lotion that might be suitable for this condition is a _____ scalp lotion. The shampoo product should be suitable for _____ scalp and hair.

21. The principal signs of dandruff are the appearance of white scales on the hair and scalp, accompanied by itching. Light rays possessing a germicidal effect that may be used to treat a dandruff condition are _____ rays. A/An _____ lamp may be used to help _____ of scalp lotions for this condition.

22. High-frequency current may be used in dandruff treatments; however, any anti-dandruff conditioners or lotions used with it cannot contain _____.

23. Conditions of alopecia may benefit from stimulation of the _____ to the germinal papilla through scalp treatments.

24. A _____ hair treatment deals with the hair _____ rather than the scalp.

25. Dry and damaged hair can be greatly improved through _____ treatments.

26. List the steps for performing a corrective hair treatment.

    1. _____

    2. _____

    3. _____

    4. _____

    5. _____

    6. _____

    7. _____

    8. _____

27. Scalp steamers, steam towels, vibrators, and scalp manipulations may all be used with hair _____. During scalp steams, the tonic is applied _____ the scalp has been steamed and _____ combing the hair into the desired style.

28. List the steps for a hair tonic treatment.

    1. _____

    2. _____

    3. _____

    4. _____

    5. _____

Chapter 13: Men's Facial Massage and Treatments

Word Review

anaphoresis	friction	phoresis
astringent	galvanic current	rolling cream
cataphoresis	general electrification	seventh cranial nerve
common carotid arteries	indirect application	tapotement
direct surface application	infrared rays	Tesla high-frequency
effleurage	iontophoresis	current
electric massager	muscles	toner
eleventh cranial nerve	percussion	ultraviolet rays
fifth cranial nerve	pétrissage	vibration

TOPIC 1: Introduction

Providing men's skin care needs is becoming an important and lucrative service in today's personal care market. A facial massage and treatment is one of the most relaxing and restful services offered in the barbershop.

1. Currently, male clients represent about _____ percent of the skin care clientele in spas and salons.

2. Historically, hot steam towels, shaves, and rolling cream facial treatments were standard customer services performed by _____ .

3. A correctly performed series of facials can produce noticeable improvement in the client's skin _____ , _____ , and _____ .

4. To perform a professional facial, barbers must be able to _____ skin conditions and recommend the most effective _____ and treatments.

TOPIC 2: Subdermal Systems and Facial Massage

1. Three of the subdermal systems associated with the performance of facial treatments are the _____ , _____ , and _____ of the head, face, and neck.

2. Fibrous tissues that have the ability to stretch, contract, and produce all body movements are _____ .

3. _____ are long, white, fibrous cords that act as message carriers from the brain and spinal column to and from all parts of the body.

4. Elastic, muscular, thick-walled blood vessels that transport blood under very high pressure are _____ .

5. _____ and treatments affect the muscles, nerves, and arteries of the head, face, and neck.

6. List the methods of stimulating muscular tissues.

   a) _____

   b) _____

   c) _____

   d) _____

   e) _____

   f) _____

   g) _____

7. When performing facial treatments, the barber is concerned with _____ muscles of the head, face, and neck. Review Table 13-1 in the textbook to complete the following chart.

Muscle	Location	Function
_____ or occipitofrontalis	_____	Broad muscle that covers the top of the skull
Frontalis	_____	Front portion of the epicranius that draws the scalp forward and causes wrinkles across the forehead
_____	Scalp	Muscle at the back part of the epicranius that draws the scalp backward
_____	Scalp	_____
_____	_____	Completely surrounds the margin of the eye socket and closes the eyelid
_____	Eyebrows	Muscle beneath the frontalis and orbicularis oculi that draws the eyebrows down and in; produces vertical lines and causes frowning
_____	_____	Covers the top of the nose, depresses the eyebrow, and causes wrinkles across the bridge of the nose; the other nasal muscles are small muscles around the nasal openings, which contract and expand the opening of the nostrils

Muscle	Location	Function
Levator labii superioris (quadratus labii superioris)	Mouth	_____ _____ _____
Depressor labii inferioris (quadratus labii inferioris)	_____	Muscle that surrounds the lower part of the lip, depressing the lower lip and drawing it a little to one side
_____	Mouth	Muscle between the upper and lower jaws; compresses the cheeks and expels air between the lips
Levator anguli oris (caninus)	Mouth	_____ _____
_____	Mouth	Situated at the tip of the chin; raises and pushes up the lower lip, causing wrinkling of the chin
_____	_____	Forms a flat band around the upper and lower lips; compresses, contracts, puckers, and wrinkles the lips
Risorius	_____	Extends from the masseter muscle to the angle of the mouth; draws the corner of the mouth out and back
_____	_____	Extends from the zygomatic bone to the angle of the mouth and elevates the lip
Triangularis	Mouth	_____ _____ _____
_____	Ears	Muscle above the ear that draws it upward
Auricularis posterior	_____	Muscle behind the ear that draws it backward

98

Muscle	Location	Function
Auricularis anterior	Ears	_____ _____
_____ _____	_____ _____	Muscles that coordinate in opening and closing the mouth and are sometimes referred to as chewing muscles
Platysma	_____ _____	Broad muscle extending from the chest and shoulder muscles to the side of the chin; responsible for depressing the lower jaw and lip
_____ _____	Neck, chest, to back of ear	Extends from the collar and chest bones to the temporal bone in back of the ear that bends and rotates the head
_____	Neck and shoulders	_____ _____

8. Stimulation to the nerves causes muscles to expand and contract; heat and moist heat on the skin causes _____ and cold causes _____.

9. List the methods used to stimulate nerves.

   a) _____

   b) _____

   c) _____

   d) _____

   e) _____

   f) _____

10. There are 12 pairs of cranial nerves and all are connected to a part of the brain surface; the cranial nerves that are of most interest when performing facial and scalp treatments are the _____, _____, and _____ cranial nerves.

11. Review Table 13-2 in the textbook to fill in the blanks.

Cranial Nerve	Name	Type	Controls
First	_____	Sensory	_____
Second	_____	Sensory	_____
Third	Oculomotor	Motor	Motion of the eye
Fourth	Trochlear	Motor	Upward/downward motion of the eye
_____	_____	(Sensory-motor)	_____
_____ _____ _____ _____ _____	Supra-orbital: affects the skin of the forehead, scalp, eyebrows, and upper eyelids Supra-trochlear: affects the skin between the eyes and upper sides of the nose Infra-trochlear: affects the membrane and skin of the nose Nasal: affects the point and lower sides of the nose Zygomatic: affects the skin of the temples, sides of the forehead, and upper part of the cheeks Infra-orbital: affects the skin of the lower eyelids, sides of the nose, upper lip, and mouth Auriculo-temporal: affects the external ear and the skin from above the temples to the top of the skull Mental: affects the skin of the lower lip and chin		
Sixth	Abducent	Motor	Motion of the eye
_____	Facial	(Sensory-motor)	_____ _____ _____
_____ _____	Posterior auricular: affects muscles behind the ears at the base of the skull Temporal: affects the muscles of the temples, sides of the forehead, eyebrows, eyelids, and upper part of the cheeks Zygomatic: affects the muscles of the upper part of the cheeks Buccal: affects the muscles of the mouth Mandibular: affects the muscles of the chin and lower lip Cervical: affects the sides of the neck		

Cranial Nerve	Name	Type	Controls
Eighth	_____	Sensory	_____
Ninth	Glossopharyngeal	Sensory-motor	Sense of taste
Tenth	Vagus	Sensory-motor	Motion and sensations of the ear, pharynx, larynx, heart, lungs, and esophagus
	Accessory	_____	_____
_____			
_____ : affects the muscles of the neck and back			
Twelfth	Hypoglossal	Motor	Motion of the tongue

12. Spinal or _____ nerves can also be affected by facial massage. Review Table 13-3 in the textbook to fill in the blanks.

Nerve	Location	Function
_____	_____	Affects the scalp as far up as the top of the head
Lesser occipital	_____	_____
	_____	
_____	_____	Affects the external ears and the areas in front and back of the ears
_____	_____	
_____	Side of the neck	Affects the front and sides of the neck as far down as the breastbone
_____		

13. An artery is a tubular vessel that is part of the circulatory system that transports blood from the heart to all parts of the body. Review Table 13-4 in the textbook to fill in the blanks provided.

Artery	Function	Arterial Branches and Blood Supply Areas
_____ _____	_____ _____ _____	Internal division: supplies the brain, eye sockets, eyelids, and forehead _____: supplies superficial parts of the head, face, and neck
External maxillary (facial artery)	_____ _____ _____	Submental: supplies chin and lower lip Inferior labial: supplies lower lip Angular: supplies side of the nose Superior labial: supplies upper lip, septum, and the wings of the nose.
Superficial temporal	_____ _____ _____ _____ _____	_____: supplies the forehead _____: supplies the crown and sides of the head Transverse facial: supplies the masseter Middle temporal: supplies the temples and eyelids Anterior auricular: supplies the anterior part of the ear
_____ _____	_____ _____ _____	_____: supplies the sternocleidomastoid muscle
Posterior _____	_____ _____ _____	Auricular artery: supplies the skin in back of the ear

14. The most important veins that serve the areas of head, neck, and chest are the internal and external _____ veins.

TOPIC 3: Theory of Massage

Facial massage involves the external manipulation of the face and requires a skillful touch.

1. The benefits of massage depend upon the _____ , _____ , and _____ of the manipulations used.

2. Massage must be performed _____ and never in a casual or _____ manner.

3. _____ skin may receive soothing, mildly stimulating, or strongly stimulating massage treatments, but _____ , inflamed skin could be damaged further by massage. Massage should be used with _____ and _____ .

4. List the conditions that may prevent the use of massage.

    a) _____

    b) _____

    c) _____

    d) _____

    e) _____

5. When massaging any part of the head, face, or neck, any pressure should be applied in an _____ direction.

6. A motor point is a point on the skin over a muscle where pressure or stimulation will cause contraction of that muscle. Review the motor points illustrated in the textbook and fill in the blanks provided on the following illustration.

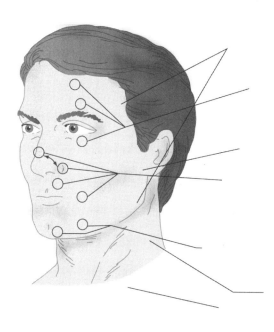
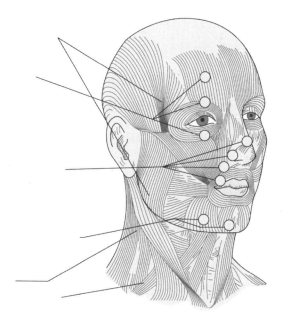

7. Review the following descriptions associated with facial massage manipulations, then identify the type of manipulation the description represents. Choices may be used more than once.

friction: deep rubbing movement

effleurage: stroking movement

pétrissage: kneading movement

vibration: rapid shaking movement

tapotement: tapping, slapping, and hacking movements

_____ performed in a slow and rhythmic manner with no pressure

_____ uses pressure while moving over an underlying structure

_____ tones the muscles and imparts a healthy glow

_____ performed with a light, firm pressure

_____ also known as tapotement

_____ may be achieved with an electric massager

_____ used for its soothing and relaxing effects

_____ involves squeezing, rolling, or light pinching

_____ gives deeper stimulation to muscles, nerves, and skin glands

_____ beneficial to circulation and glandular activity of the skin

_____ the most stimulating massage manipulation

_____ should never exceed a few seconds' duration on any one spot

8. Skillfully applied massage influences the structures and functions of the body, but its immediate effect is first noticed on the _____ .

9. List the physiological benefits of massage.

a) _____

b) _____

c) _____

d) _____

e) _____

f) _____

g) _____

h) _____

10. In massage, an even tempo or rhythm induces _____.

11. Once massage manipulations have begun, _____ or _____ should remain on the skin at all times.

12. When it becomes necessary to remove the hands from the face, gently _____ the hands from the skin.

13. Massage movements are directed from the _____ toward the _____ of a muscle to avoid damage to muscular tissues; apply _____ pressure on the motor points of the face.

14. Order the following list of massage movements as presented in the textbook.

_____ Manipulate fingers across the forehead with a circular movement.

_____ Manipulate the temples, and then the front and back of the ears, with a wide circular movement

_____ Apply cleansing cream lightly over the face with stroking, spreading, and circulatory movements.

_____ Stroke fingers upward along sides of nose.

_____ Stroke fingers above and below lower jawbone from the chin to the ear. Manipulate fingers from under the chin and neck to the back of the ears and up to the temples.

_____ Stroke fingers across forehead with up-and-down movements.

_____ Gently stroke both thumbs across upper lip.

_____ Apply a circular movement over sides of nose, and use a light, stroking movement around the eyes.

_____ Manipulate fingers from the corners of the mouth to the cheeks and temples with a rotary movement. Manipulate fingers along the lower jaw from the tip of the chin to the ear using the same technique.

15. What technique should be used when facial hair prevents using an upward direction of massage movements? _____
_____

TOPIC 4: Equipment for Massage Treatments

1. Appliances that can be used to enhance the facial treatment service are: _____ or _____, _____, _____, _____, and _____ rays.

2. An _____ transmits vibrations through the barber's hand to the client's skin and muscles.

3. A _____ helps to stimulate, cleanse, and lightly exfoliate the skin; no _____ should be applied and it is not _____ for use on inflamed or acne-prone skin.

4. _____ are electrical devices that produce and project a moist, uniform steam for the purposes of softening, _____, warming, inducing the flow of _____ and _____, and providing an _____ effect on the skin.

5. Facial treatments performed with electric facial machines are a form of _____.

6. The electrical currents used in electrotherapy are: _____, _____, _____, and _____ currents; some _____ can generate all four currents.

7. Electrical modality machines require an _____ to apply and direct the current to the skin.

8. Except for the _____ modality, each of the currents requires two electrodes, one positive and one negative.

9. A positive electrode, or _____ is red; a negative electrode, or _____ is black.

10. The high-frequency, or _____ current is characterized by a high rate of _____ and is sometimes called the violet ray because of its color.

11. The primary actions of the high-frequency current are _____ and _____; the effects are either _____ or _____, depending on the method of application.

12. Electrodes for high-frequency current are made of _____ or _____.

13. All high-frequency treatments should begin with a _____ current that is gradually _____ to the required strength for no longer than _____.

14. When performing electrotherapy treatments, the barber and the client must avoid contact with _____ or _____.

15. List the ways in which high-frequency can benefit the skin.

    a) _____

    b) _____

    c) _____

    d) _____

    e) _____

    f) _____

    g) _____

16. Fill in the blanks to complete the applications, procedures, and benefits associated with using Tesla high-frequency current.

Method	Application	Procedure	Benefits
Direct	Can be used on clean, _____ skin, over facial creams, and over gauze for a sparking effect	_____ _____ Adjust rheostat to proper setting. Place _____ on glass electrode. Apply electrode _____ _____; begin at the forehead. _____ electrode over skin in circular upward movements on the neck towards the jaw, cheeks, chin, nose, and forehead. Remove from skin by placing index finger over the _____ and then remove electrode. Turn power switch off.	Produces _____ effects on the skin
Indirect	Performed with the client holding the wire glass electrode between both hands; power is turned on _____ the client is holding the electrode and turned off _____ the electrode is removed from the client's hand.	Apply _____ to client's face. Instruct client to hold the wire glass electrode with both hands. Place the fingers of one hand on client's _____. With the opposite hand, turn the high-frequency current on to a low setting. Using both hands, perform tapping motions in a systematic manner over the client's face. To discontinue the high-frequency service, the barber _____ _____ _____.	Produces _____ effects on the skin; ideal for aging and sallow skin
General electrification	Charges the client's body with electricity	Client holds a _____ electrode while massage is performed by the barber.	Produces calming, sedative, or _____ effects

17. Glass electrodes are cleansed by wiping with a soap and water solution and by placing the end only into a _____ solution for 20 minutes.

18. Electrodes should _____ be placed in an ultraviolet-ray sanitizer or autoclave.

19. _____ use a skin or scalp lotion containing alcohol prior to a high-frequency treatment.

20. The _____ machine converts the oscillating current received from an outlet into a _____ current so that the electrons then flow continuously in the same direction.

21. A relaxation response can be regulated to target specific nerve endings in the epidermis using _____ current.

22. Galvanic current produces chemical reactions, or _____, and ionic reactions, or _____, in the skin that are beneficial for _____ or _____ skin problems.

23. The most popular electrodes for the galvanic machine are the _____ and the _____ roller; to make proper contact, each electrode must be covered with cotton and the client must hold the _____ pole electrode.

24. desincrustation is used for deep pore cleansing. Fill in the blanks to complete the steps for the procedure.

    1. _____ .

    2. Instruct client to remove any _____ from the hand that will hold the electrode. Cover the _____ electrode with a moistened sponge or piece of cotton.

    3. Prepare the desincrustation electrode (_____ electrode) with a dampened sponge or cotton pad.

    4. Dip the electrode into the desincrustation solution and apply the electrode to the client's forehead; turn the switch to negative and set at _____ micro-amps.

    5. Gently glide and rotate the electrode over the facial areas that are _____; reduce the current back to zero before moving the electrode to another section of the face.

    6. When finished, turn the machine off and remove the _____ .

25. Iontophoresis means the introduction of ions; galvanic current is used to apply _____ solutions into the deeper layers of the skin.

26. The client holds an electrode with the _____ charge.

27. _____ is the process of forcing chemical solutions into unbroken skin by way of a galvanic current.

28. The process of ionic penetration takes place in two forms: _____ and _____ . Cataphoresis uses the positive pole to introduce acid-pH products into the skin, and anaphoresis uses the negative pole to force alkaline-pH products into the skin.

29. The _____ machine is an electronic vacuum that is used to spray micro-crystals across the skin's surface.

30. _____ are used to impart light therapy treatments to the skin.

31. Infrared, ultraviolet, white, blue, and red rays are used to produce different effects through the use of _____ .

32. Ultraviolet ray lamps are used to treat acne, tinea, seborrhea, and dandruff conditions for their _____ effects; benefits of the shorter rays are obtained when the lamp is placed within _____ of the skin.

33. Infrared rays produce a soothing and beneficial type of heat that extends into the tissues of the body. List the effects of infrared rays on the skin.

    a) _____

    b) _____

    c) _____

    d) _____

    e) _____

34. The infrared ray lamp is operated at an average distance of _____ .

35. Fill in the blanks to complete the suggested list of safety precautions for using electrical equipment.

    a) _____ any appliances when they are not being used.

    b) Study _____ before using any electrical equipment.

    c) Keep all wires, plugs, and equipment in a _____ condition.

    d) _____ all electrical equipment frequently.

    e) Avoid _____ electric cords.

    f) _____ all electrodes properly.

    g) Protect the _____ at all times.

    h) Do not touch any _____ while using electrical appliances.

    i) Do not handle electrical equipment with _____ hands.

    j) Do not allow _____ to touch metal surfaces when electrical treatments are being performed.

    k) Do not leave the room when the client is attached to any _____ device.

    l) Do not attempt to clean around an electric outlet when equipment is _____ .

    m) Do not touch two metallic objects at the same time while _____ to an electric current.

    n) Do not use any electrical equipment without first obtaining full _____ in its care and use.

TOPIC 5: Facial Treatments

1. The barber does not treat skin _____ , but should be able to perform _____ or _____ facial treatments.

2. _____ treatments are intended to help maintain the health of facial skin.

3. _____ treatments are used to correct skin conditions such as _____ , oiliness, _____ , aging lines, and minor acne.

4. List the ways in which facials are beneficial to the skin and body.

   a) _____

   b) _____

   c) _____

   d) _____

   e) _____

   f) _____

   g) _____

   h) _____

   i) _____

   j) _____

5. Preparations or products used in facial treatments include facial _____ , _____ , _____ , _____ , _____ , _____ , and _____ .

6. There are _____ basic skin types; skin types are based on the amount of _____ that is produced in the _____ from the _____ glands.

7. The basic skin types are _____ , _____ , _____ , and _____ .

8. Any skin types can be _____ to products, irritation, or the environment.

9. Choose from one of the four skin types to determine the correct answer for the following skin characteristics or descriptions.

   _____ needs extra care

   _____ has a good water-to-oil balance

   _____ characterized by excess sebum production

   _____ has an oily T-zone and dry cheeks

   _____ follicle size is larger

   _____ moisturizers and humectants can help

   _____ requires more cleansing and exfoliation

110

_____ follicles are an average size

_____ does not produce enough oil

_____ maintenance and preservation is the goal

_____ water-based products work best for this type

_____ a water-based hydrator may help balance this type

_____ can be oily and dry

10. Wrinkles are depressions in the skin that develop from repeated muscle actions moving in the same direction. Fill in the blanks to complete the list of other factors that influence the formation of wrinkles.

   a) _____ of elastic skin _____ due to tension or relaxation of the facial muscles

   b) _____ of the skin tissue as a result of aging

   c) excessive _____ of the skin

   d) _____ facial care

11. A knowledge of skin types and conditions helps the barber to perform an accurate skin analysis. List the guidelines for performing a skin analysis.

   1. _____

   2. _____

   3. _____

   4. _____

12. The type of _____ treatment will determine the products needed to complete the procedure.

13. Three essential facial products are _____, _____, and _____.

14. _____ are available as face washes, lotions, and creams for all types of skin and skin conditions. Match the appropriate type of cleanser with the following descriptions.

_____ water-based emulsions

_____ water-based products of a neutral or slightly acidic pH

_____ oil-based emulsions

_____ effective for oily and combination skin

_____ dissolve dirt and heavy makeup

_____ for normal and combination skin

_____ contain emollients or oils

a) face washes

b) cleansing lotions

c) cleansing cream

111

15. _____, _____, and _____ are used after cleansing and prior to the application of a moisturizer; these tonic lotions vary in _____, _____ content, and _____.

16. Match the appropriate tonic with the following descriptions. Descriptions may describe more than one type of tonic.

_____ used for oily skin

_____ temporarily tighten the skin

_____ have the lowest alcohol content

_____ contain up to 35 percent alcohol

_____ used for dry, mature, and sensitive skin

_____ tone or tighten the skin

_____ used for normal and combination skin

_____ used for acne-prone skin

_____ 4 to 15 percent alcohol content

a) fresheners

b) toners

c) astringents

17. _____ are formulated to add moisture to the skin and are available for various skin types in _____ and _____ formulations.

18. _____ are used to physically rub or remove dead cells from the skin surface.

19. _____ and _____ draw impurities out of pores, tighten, _____, hydrate, soothe, and nourish the skin, depending on the ingredients.

20. Clay masks stimulate circulation, contract the skin pores, and absorb _____.

21. Paraffin wax masks employ the _____ application method.

22. _____ creams are creams, lotions, or oils that provide slip during a massage.

23. _____ cream is a thick, smooth, facial cleanser that is rolled off with a firm, stroking motion.

24. List the order in which the skin care products are used during the facial treatments, as indicated in the textbook.

1. _____

2. _____

3. _____

4. _____

5. _____

6. _____

7. _____

8. _____

25. When choosing men's skin care products, creams should be simple, _____, and absorbent with a _____ finish; men also prefer simpler routines and _____ products.

26. As a general rule, products that are _____ in the barbershop should be used for services performed within the shop.

TOPIC 6: Facial Procedures

1. The basic facial is sometimes known as the _____ facial. Fill in the blanks where needed to complete the procedural steps of this facial.

    1. Arrange all necessary supplies in a convenient location.

    2. Drape the client and engage in _____.

    3. Make _____ selection.

    4. Place a _____ between the client's head and the headrest. Adjust the headrest and recline the hydraulic chair. Make sure the client is comfortable.

    5. Protect the client's _____ with a towel or cap.

    6. Wash your hands.

    7. Apply _____ over the face, using stroking and rotary movements.

    8. Remove the cleansing cream with a warm, damp towel.

    9. Apply two or three _____ to open pores and loosen imbedded dirt and oils.

    10. Reapply cleansing cream to the skin with the fingertips.

    11. Gently _____ the face, using continuous and rhythmic movements. Wipe off excess cleansing cream with a warm towel.

    12. Apply an _____ product and lightly massage over the skin.

    13. Apply steam towel. Wipe off excess product until the skin is free of exfoliating _____.

    14. Gently wipe _____ or astringent over the face, and then pat dry.

    15. Apply mask or pack and allow to dry.

    16. Apply tepid to warm towel to _____ mask or pack. Wipe off the product until free of mask or pack.

    17. Gently wipe toner or astringent over the face and pat dry.

    18. Apply a light coat of _____ using the effleurage movement.

    19. Apply a light dusting of talc if the client desires it. Remove any excess.

    20. Slowly raise the hydraulic chair and _____ client to a sitting position.

    21. Discard all disposable supplies and materials.

    22. Wipe containers and _____. Store in appropriate place.

    23. _____ all non-disposable implements and tools.

    24. Wash and sanitize your hands.

2. All products should be removed from their containers with a _____ . Dipping the fingers into products may _____ the preparation.

3. List some points that should be remembered when performing a facial.

   a) _____

   b) _____

   c) _____

   d) _____

   e) _____

4. Fill in the blanks to complete the list of actions to avoid when performing a facial.

   a) harming or _____ the skin

   b) excessive or rough _____

   c) getting _____ in the client's eyes

   d) using towels that are too _____

   e) _____ into the client's face

   f) being careless or _____

   g) showing _____ in the client's skin problems or conversation

   h) leaving _____ product on the skin

   i) excessive _____ that does not facilitate client relaxation

   j) _____ the chair to obtain materials or supplies

   k) having heavy, rough, or cold _____

5. An _____ may be used during a vibratory facial, but _____ contact with the client's skin should be avoided.

6. Fill in the blanks to complete the explanation for holding the electric massager during a vibratory facial.

   _____ of the barber's hands need to be used. The right-handed barber attaches the massager to his right hand. The left hand is placed on the client's _____ . Next, the barber places his right hand on top of his left and the _____ travel through his left hand to the client's skin. Direct contact with the barber's right hand can be made to less _____ areas such as the forehead and jaw line, but pressure still needs to be avoided.

7. The vibrator should never be used when there is a known _____ of the _____ or in cases of _____ , _____ , or skin inflammations.

114

8. When performing massage movements with an electric massager, begin at the client's left nostril with up-and-down movements along the side of the _____. Slide the fingers along the upper _____ area, then toward the center of the _____. Use rotary movements at the _____ and along the jaw line to the tip of the chin. Work from the chin back to the temple and around the left _____, then back over the jawbone, toward the center of the _____ below the chin. Repeat on the right side of the face.

9. Fill in the blanks where needed to list the steps of the vibratory facial procedure.

    1. Prepare the client as for a _____ facial.

    2. Apply steam towels.

    3. Apply _____ cream.

    4. Administer the massage using the _____.

    5. Apply _____ cream with light hand manipulations.

    6. Remove cleansing cream with a warm towel.

    7. Follow with a mild witch hazel _____.

    8. Apply one or two cool towels.

    9. Apply a _____ face lotion.

    10. Dry thoroughly and apply powder if desired.

10. Fill in the blanks to list the rules for using an electric massager.

    a) Regulate the number of vibrations to avoid _____.

    b) Do not use the vibrator for too long in any one spot.

    c) Vary the amount of _____ in accordance with the results desired.

    d) Do not use a vibrator over the _____ to avoid discomfort.

    e) Use slow, light vibrations for a short time for soothing and relaxing effects.

    f) For stimulating effects, give light vibrations of _____ speed and time.

    g) To reduce fatty tissues, give moderate, fast vibrations with _____ pressure.

11. The type of facial massage most often identified with the barbershop is the _____ facial, which is designed to cleanse and stimulate the skin.

12. The rolling cream facial should be recommended only to clients with _____, _____, or _____ skin; it should not be performed on skin that is _____, _____, _____, or _____ in texture.

13. Fill in the blanks to complete the steps for the rolling cream facial.

    1. Prepare the client.

    2. Moderately steam the face with two or three warm towels.

3. Apply dabs of _____ to the chin, cheeks, and forehead. Dampen the fingertips of both hands with _____ and spread the cream evenly over the face and neck with a smooth, stroking movement.

4. Massage the face and neck with _____ rotary, stroking, and rubbing movements with the cushion tips of the fingers until most of the cream has rolled off.

5. Apply a small amount of _____ to the face and neck, using lighter manipulations.

6. Remove the cream with a warm towel.

7. Apply witch hazel _____ to the face and neck with one or more hot towels, following with one or two _____ towels to close the pores.

8. Apply astringent lotion. Dry and powder the face and neck.

9. Finish as for a basic facial.

14. The objective of a facial for dry skin is to help _____ it; dry skin facials can be performed using _____, _____ current, or _____ current.

15. Fill in the blanks to complete the steps used to perform a dry skin facial using infrared rays.

    1. Prepare the client as for a basic facial.

    2. Apply cleansing cream; remove cream with a warm, moist towel.

    3. Sponge the face with a mild _____ lotion.

    4. Apply _____ cream.

    5. Apply _____ oil or eye cream over and under the eyes.

    6. Apply lubricating oil over the neck.

    7. Cover the client's _____ with cotton pads moistened with witch hazel or a non-alcoholic freshener.

    8. Expose the face and neck to _____ rays for not more than _____ minutes.

    9. Perform massage _____ three to five times.

    10. Remove massage cream and oil with tissues or with a warm, moist towel.

    11. Apply _____ lotion for dry skin. Blot the face dry with tissues or a towel.

    12. Apply _____.

    13. Complete and clean up as for a basic facial.

16. Explain the method used to break the path of the infrared rays on the skin. _____

_____

17. The total exposure time when using infrared rays should not exceed _____.

18. When giving a dry skin facial with galvanic current, many of the steps are the same as the procedure using infrared rays. List the steps that are different.

    a) _____

    b) _____

    c) _____

    d) _____

19. When giving a dry skin facial using indirect high-frequency current, many of the steps are the same as the procedure using infrared rays. List the steps that are different.

    a) _____

    b) _____

    _____

    c) _____

20. Oily skin and/or blackheads are caused by hardened masses of sebum formed in the ducts of the sebaceous glands. Fill in the blanks to complete the steps to perform a facial for oily skin and blackheads.

    1. Prepare the client as for a basic facial.

    2. Apply _____ lotion and remove it with a warm, moist towel or facial sponges.

    3. Place moistened eye pads on the client's eyes, then analyze the skin under a magnifying lamp.

    4. _____ the face with three or four moist, warm towels or a facial steamer to open the pores.

    5. Wear _____, cover your fingertips with _____, and gently press out blackheads.

    6. Sponge the face with _____.

    7. (Optional: Cover the client's eyes with pads moistened with a mild astringent. Apply _____ light over the skin for 3 to 5 minutes.)

    8. Apply appropriate _____ cream and perform manipulations.

    9. Remove cream with a warm, moist towel, cotton pads, or facial sponges.

    10. Apply _____ lotion to the face and neck.

    11. Apply _____ or protective lotion according to skin type.

    12. Complete and clean up as for basic facial procedure.

21. Acne is a disorder of the sebaceous glands and serious cases require medical direction; if the client is under medical care, the role of the barber is to perform facial treatments as _____ by the client's physician.

22. The treatment of acne conditions, with a prescribed treatment plan for the barber to follow, should be limited to the following.

a) _____

b) _____

c) _____

d) _____

23. Barbers should wear _____ when performing the acne facial and should use _____ materials.

24. Many of the steps used for the acne facial are the same as those used in the facial for oily skin. What important caution is noted in the acne facial procedure? _____

_____

25. A _____ mask can be used for extremely dry, parched, and scaly skin that is prevalent during dry, hot, or windy weather. The type of light therapy that may be used during this procedure is an _____ lamp.

Chapter 14: Shaving and Facial Hair Design

Word Review

backhand

changeable-blade razor

close shaving

conventional straight razor

cutting stroke

freehand

neck shave

once-over shave

reverse backhand

reverse freehand

second-time-over shave

styptic powder

TOPIC 1: Introduction

A full facial shave, complete with hot towels, lotions, and massage, is one of the most relaxing yet rejuvenating services that men can enjoy in the barbershop.

1. Today's barbers need to master _____ skills to ensure the longevity of the profession.

2. Shaving is an art that requires careful attention, skill, and _____ to perfect.

TOPIC 2: Fundamentals of Shaving

1. The objective of shaving is to remove the visible part of facial and neck hair without _____ to the skin.

2. Professional barbers use a _____ or _____ straight razor and warm lather when shaving a client.

3. The application of _____ is a standard procedure in preparing the beard for shaving; however, some clients may not _____ a hot towel on their skin.

4. Variables that barbers must consider before proceeding with the shave service include individual characteristics such as hair _____, hair _____, and product _____.

5. Fill in the blanks to complete sanitation and safety precautions associated with shaving.

   1. Always _____ tools before using.

   2. Once the client is in position for the shave, _____ the chair.

   3. Use a _____ touch and forward _____ motion with the _____ of the blade leading.

   4. Always observe the hair growth pattern and shave _____ it, not _____ it.

   5. Heavy beard growth may require more lathering and _____.

   6. Lather _____ the grain gently to place the facial hair in a position to be shaved.

119

7. Lather should be applied _____ to the areas to be shaved and lather should be replaced as necessary.

8. The fingers of the hand opposite the hand holding the razor should be kept _____ in order to grasp, stretch, and hold the skin firmly during the shave service.

9. Do not use _____ towels on skin that is chapped or blistered from heat or cold, or skin that is thin and sensitive.

10. When astringents are too harsh for sensitive skin, _____ or toners should be used.

11. Do not serve clients who have an infection in the area to be shaved because doing so could _____ or to the barber.

12. Curly facial hair requires special care to minimize the occurrence of _____; avoid shaving too close or with too much _____.

13. Take special precautions when shaving sensitive areas such as beneath the lower lip, the lower part of the neck, and around the _____.

14. Use styptic powder on a cotton swab or pledget on small cuts and nicks; never use a styptic _____ or other astringent that will come into contact with another person's face.

15. Keep the skin _____ while shaving.

16. Some states may require the use of _____ while shaving a client.

17. Follow through with _____ from one shaving area to another; do not stop short.

18. Some states prohibit the use of _____ straight razors and allow only changeable-blade razors.

TOPIC 3: Razor Positions and Strokes

1. Label the parts of the razor in the following illustration.

2. The correct angle of cutting the beard with a straight razor is called the _____.

3. To achieve the best cutting stroke, the razor must glide over the surface at an angle _____ , with the _____ of the razor leading.

4. When opening the razor, the _____ of the razor's blade is held between the thumb and index finger of the dominant hand.

5. When closing the razor, the handle is pivoted or moved to the _____ .

6. List the four razor positions and strokes used in barbering.

   1. _____

   2. _____

   3. _____

   4. _____

7. List the three razor positions and strokes used in facial shaving.

   1. _____

   2. _____

   3. _____

8. Each of the four razor positions and strokes requires knowing _____ to use a particular shaving stroke; _____ to hold the razor for each stroke and the position of the right and left hands _____ ; and how to _____ the razor.

9. Identify the four shaving positions and strokes in the following photographs.

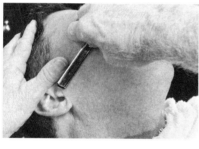

_____

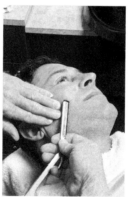

_____

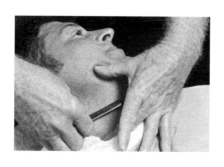

_____

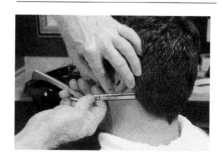

_____

10. Number the shaving areas in the following illustration. Next, draw the directional arrows for each area. Then, shade the areas in which a freehand stroke is used to shave the face.

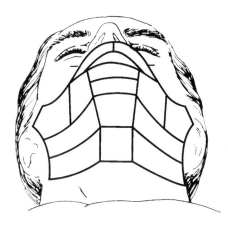

11. In which shaving areas is the freehand position and stroke used? _____, _____, _____, _____, _____, and _____.

12. The backhand position and stroke is used in shaving areas _____, _____, _____, and _____.

13. The reverse freehand stroke is used in shaving areas _____, _____, _____, and _____.

14. When might the reverse backhand stroke be used? _____
_____

TOPIC 4: The Shave Service

1. A professional shave consists of _____, _____, and _____.

2. _____ cleans the face, softens the hair, holds the hair in an upright position, and creates a smooth, flat surface for the razor.

3. _____ the face helps to soften the hair cuticle, provides lubrication by stimulating the action of the oil glands, and relaxes the client.

4. Why should mustaches be trimmed and shaped prior to the shave service? _____
_____

5. Fill in the blanks where necessary to complete the steps used to prepare a client for a shave service.

    1. Seat the client comfortably in the chair.

    2. Ask the client to loosen his collar, drape towel _____, and position the cape over the client's clothing.

    3. Change the _____ and adjust it to the proper height.

    4. Lower, adjust, and _____ the chair to the proper height and level.

    5. Wash your hands with soap and warm water and dry them thoroughly.

122

6. Lay a second clean towel _____ across the client's chest.

7. Tuck towel into the _____ of the drape, then tuck a paper strip into the neckband.

8. Prepare and apply a _____ towel.

9. Prepare lather and transfer into your hand.

10. Remove steam towel and spread lather evenly over the bearded areas of the face and neck to be shaved using _____ movements.

11. Start at the _____ and work up toward the right side of the face; repeat on left side.

12. Test the _____ of the second steam towel against your _____, then apply over the lather and mold the towel to conform to the face.

13. Prepare and _____ the razor while the steam towel is on the client's face.

14. Remove the steam towel and wipe the lather off in one operation. Re-lather the beard in preparation for _____ and wipe lather from your hands.

6. As the right hand holds and strokes the razor, the fingers of the left hand _____ the skin to be shaved.

7. How is the once-over shave performed? _____
_____

8. Performing a second-time-over shave removes any rough or unshaven spots and may be considered a form of _____.

9. Close shaving is the practice of shaving the beard _____ of the hair during the _____ phase of the shave.

10. Close shaving may irritate the skin and lead to _____ or _____.

11. The final steps of a shave service require attention to a number of important details. Fill in the blanks where necessary to complete the steps for finishing the shave service.

1. Apply facial cream or _____ lotion using _____ movements.

2. Apply a _____ warm towel over the face.

3. Remove the towel from the face.

4. Apply a _____ or other mild astringent.

5. Remove the towel from the client's chest and position yourself behind the chair.

6. Spread the towel over the client's face and _____.

7. Wrap a clean, dry towel around your hand.

8. Sprinkle _____ on the towel and apply evenly to the face.

9. Slowly raise the chair to an upright position.

10. Perform a _____ if requested.

11. Comb the hair neatly as desired.

12. Wipe off loose hair, lather, or powder from the client's _____ , _____ , and _____ . Remove draping.

12. Barbers use towel wraps for cleansing and drying the face, for applying powder to the face, and for removing traces of _____ , _____ , and _____ from the face, neck, and forehead.

13. The _____ involves shaving the neckline on both sides of the neck, below the ears, and across the nape if desired or necessary.

14. When performing a neck shave, shave the right side using a _____ stroke, the left side using a _____ , and a freehand stroke in the nape area.

15. There are many reasons why a client may find fault with a shave procedure. List ten of the most common.

1. _____

2. _____

3. _____

4. _____

5. _____

6. _____

7. _____

8. _____

9. _____

10. _____

TOPIC 5: Facial Hair Design

1. Choosing a suitable mustache design depends on the client's _____ , _____ , and personal taste.

2. The size of the mustache should correspond to the size of the _____ .

3. What are some important facial characteristics that help to determine the choice of a mustache design? _____
_____

4. Fill in the blanks to complete the following guidelines associated with mustache design and proportion.

   a) large, coarse facial features: _____ looking mustache

   b) prominent nose: _____ to large mustache

c) long, narrow face: narrow to _____ mustache

d) extra-large mouth: _____ mustache

e) extra-small mouth: _____ to _____ mustache

f) smallish, regular features: smaller, _____ mustache

g) wide mouth with prominent upper lip: heavier handlebar or large, _____ mustache

h) round face with regular features: _____ mustache

i) square face with prominent features: heavier, _____ mustache with ends slightly curving _____ .

5. List the steps for performing a mustache trim.

   1. _____

   2. _____

   3. _____

      _____

   4. _____

   5. _____

6. Additional mustache services include waxing mustache ends, _____ with temporary color, or _____ .

7. Beards and goatees can be used to _____ facial features or to correlate the _____ of the head, face, and body.

8. The correct shaping or redesign of the beard can _____ pleasant facial features, _____ less desirable ones, and _____ flaws.

9. Beard design and trimming is usually performed with a combination of the _____ , _____ , _____ , _____ , and _____ .

10. Fill in the blanks where necessary to complete the steps for performing a beard trim.

    1. Drape the client as for a haircut service.

    2. Consult with the client as to his desired design of the beard.

    3. Draw in the beard design with an eyebrow pencil _____ .

    4. Adjust the _____ .

    5. Place a towel underneath the client's _____ .

    6. Trim _____ hair with shear-over-comb or _____ technique.

    7. Create a _____ with the outliner. Start in the _____ directly under the chin and outline the under part of the beard.

8. Outline the cheek and upper areas of the beard, blending with the _____ area.

9. Use the shear-over-comb technique to taper and blend the beard from the _____ areas up to just under the bottom lip, mustache, and cheek areas.

10. Apply steam towel, _____ areas to be shaved, shave carefully at the outline, and wipe clean.

11. Return client to sitting position.

12. Wipe off any remaining lather or pencil marks. Apply aftershave or _____ lotion.

13. Trim and blend the _____. Follow with razor work as necessary.

14. _____ and retouch the beard with shears and outliner wherever necessary.

15. Style or cut the hair as needed for a finished look.

11. Clippers are effective for creating a beard design that is _____ overall.

12. Clipper-cut beard trims are most successful on beards with even _____ and _____.

13. Explain how to choose detachable-blade sizes for beard trimming with the clipper. _____
_____
_____

14. _____ are usually used in the final trimming step of a beard trim.

Chapter 15: Men's Haircutting and Styling

Word Review

angle	freehand clipper cutting	reference points
arching technique	freehand shear cutting	rolling the comb out
blow-dry styling	freehand slicing	shear-over-comb
clipper-over-comb	guide	shear-point tapering
crest	hairlocking	stationary guide
crown	horizontal	tapered
cutting above the fingers	layers	tension
cutting below the fingers	outlining	texturizing
design line	over-direction	thinning
diagonal	parietal ridge	traveling guide
elevation	parting	vertical
envisioning	projection	weight line
facial shapes	razor rotation	
fingers-and-shear	razor-over-comb	

TOPIC 1: Introduction

The art of haircutting involves individualized and precise designing, cutting, and shaping of the hair. In order to perform the art of haircutting successfully, barbers must be at ease using a variety of tools, implements, techniques, and methods.

1. A _____ is the foundation of a good _____.

2. A haircut and style should _____ the client's strong features and _____ the weaker ones.

3. The client's wishes, _____, lifestyle, _____, facial contour, _____, neckline, and hair _____ are all factors that must be considered when designing the haircut and style.

TOPIC 2: Client Consultation

1. A client _____ helps to eliminate guesswork about the haircut or style.

2. List some basic questions that barbers might ask a client before beginning a haircut.

   a) _____

   b) _____

   c) _____

   d) _____

3. What is envisioning? _____

_____

TOPIC 3: Basic Principles of Haircutting and Styling

1. Every haircut is a representation and _____ of the barber's work.

2. _____ is defined as the artistic cutting and dressing of hair to best fit the client's physical needs and personality.

3. Facial shapes are determined by the position and prominence of the _____.

4. The seven general facial shapes are:

   1. _____

   2. _____

   3. _____

   4. _____

   5. _____

   6. _____

   7. _____

5. Fill in the blanks to match the characteristic with the correct facial shape listed in question 4.

   a) _____ face shape needs to be shortened

   b) _____ goal is to slim the face

   c) _____ shape is narrow at the top, wide at the bottom

   d) _____ considered the ideal face shape

   e) _____ over-wide cheekbones and narrow jaw line

   f) _____ needs filling out at the temples and chin

   g) _____ goal is to minimize angular features at the forehead

6. The shape of the _____ influences the profile, and the _____ can influence the appropriateness of a haircut or style.

7. Review the following characteristics of profiles and nose shapes, then fill in the blank with the correct type.

   a) _____ profiles that are usually the most balanced

   b) _____ profiles that require minimizing the bulge of the forehead

   c) _____ examples include a hooked nose, large nose, or pointed nose

   d) _____ profiles that require concealment of a short, receding forehead

   e) _____ size and/or heavy features are not an issue for this nose shape

   f) _____ profiles that need balance at the forehead to offset a chin that juts forward

   g) _____ minimizes a receding chin.

8. Long necks are minimized when the hair is left _____ or _____.

9. Short necks can look longer with a _____ neckline.

TOPIC 4: Fundamentals of Haircutting

1. The fundamental principles of haircutting include the _____, basic _____ used in haircutting, and haircutting _____.

2. Why does hair respond differently in different areas of the head? _____
_____

3. The sections of the head include the _____, _____, _____, _____, _____, _____, _____, and _____.

4. The temporal section is part of the _____; it is also known as the _____, _____, or _____ region of the head.

5. What are reference points? _____
_____

6. Review the following descriptions, then match them with the correct section of the head. Choices may be used more than once.

    _____ protrudes at the base of the skull   a) parietal ridge

    _____ also known as the crest   b) occipital bone

    _____ begins where the head curves away from the nape   c) apex

    _____ also known as the horseshoe or hatband area

    _____ highest point on the top of the head

    _____ widest section of the head

    _____ transition area from the top to the front, sides, and back

7. Label the sections of the head in the following figures.

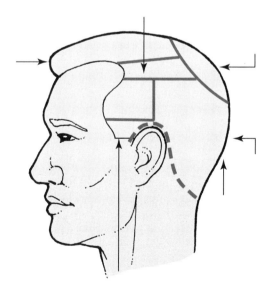
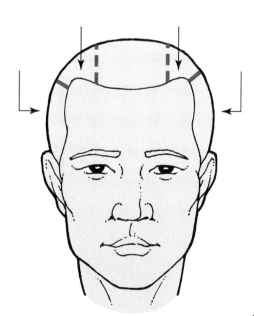

129

8. The three types of straight lines used in haircutting are _____ , _____ , and _____ lines.

9. Review the following descriptions and characteristics of lines, then fill in the blank with the correct type of line. Answers may be used more than once.

a) _____ lines that are perpendicular to the floor

b) _____ lines that are parallel to the horizon

c) _____ lines that have a slanted direction

d) _____ lines that direct the eye up and down

e) _____ cutting lines that build weight

f) _____ used to remove weight within the cut

g) _____ used to create sloped lines at the perimeter

h) _____ used to create a one-length look

i) _____ used to create a blunt cut

j) _____ allows projection of the hair at higher elevations

k) _____ used to create layers within a cut

l) _____ may refer to finger placement when stacking at the perimeter

10. Angles can refer to the _____ at which the hair is held for cutting or to the _____ when cutting a section of hair.

11. The angle or degree at which a section of hair is held from the head for cutting, relative to where it grows, is called _____ .

12. Elevation is also known as _____ ; it is the result of lifting the hair section above _____ and is usually described in terms of _____ .

13. Review the following descriptions and identify them as being characteristic of 0 elevation, 45 degrees, or 90 degrees.

a) _____ medium elevation

b) _____ high elevation

c) _____ low elevation

d) _____ requires a traveling guide

e) _____ produces weight at the perimeter

f) _____ creates layered ends or stacking

g) _____ produces maximum length at the perimeter

h) _____ common elevation used in men's haircutting

i) _____ used to achieve the standard blunt cut

130

j) _____ hair is held straight out from where it grows

k) _____ hair is held straight down in natural fall

l) _____ also known as graduation

m) _____ produces layered, tapered, and blended effects

n) _____ used to create uniform or tapered layers

14. A _____ is a smaller section of hair parted off from a larger section or subsection.

15. The outer perimeter line of the haircut is called the _____.

16. A _____ is a cut that is made so that subsequent sections of hair can be measured and cut.

17. Guides are either _____ or _____.

18. The type of guide that is used to maintain length in one section while subsequent partings are brought to it for cutting is called a _____.

19. A _____ moves along a section of hair and makes use of the previous guide to cut a subsequent parting of hair.

20. Layers are produced by cutting the hair at elevations higher than _____.

21. When the hair conforms to the shape of the head and is shorter at the nape and longer in the top area, it is considered to be _____.

22. A _____ refers to the heaviest perimeter area of a 0-elevation or 45-degree cut.

23. Creating special, wispy, or spiky effects within a haircut are forms of _____.

24. _____ is the amount of pressure applied while combing and holding a section of hair for cutting.

25. Removing excess bulk from the hair is called _____.

26. _____ is the marking or finishing of the outer perimeter of a haircut along the hairline.

27. A length increase in the design can be achieved if the hair is _____.

28. Arranging the hair in a particular style that is appropriately suited to the cut is called _____.

29. Hairstyle trends tend to be _____.

30. Barbers should become proficient in the _____ in order to adapt to whatever the current trend may be.

TOPIC 5: Haircutting Techniques

1. List the cutting techniques used in barbering.

   a) _____

   b) _____

   c) _____

   d) _____

   e) _____

   f) _____

   g) _____

2. Almost every haircutting procedure requires a combination of _____ and _____.

3. List the three basic methods for using the fingers-and-shear technique.

   1. _____

   2. _____

   3. _____

4. When cutting on top of the fingers to create layers in the top section of a haircut, the fingers and shear are positioned _____ or _____ to the parting.

5. When cutting on top of the fingers to create layers in the side section of a haircut, the fingers and shear are positioned _____ or _____ to the floor and parallel to the parting.

6. When cutting below the fingers to create a design line in the nape section, the fingers and shears are positioned _____.

7. When the process of rolling the comb out is used to position the hair to be cut, the technique being used is the _____ technique.

8. The _____ technique is helpful when tapering in the nape, behind-the-ear, around-the-ear, and sideburn areas of a cut.

9. The _____ blade of the shears and the _____ should be aligned when cutting with the shear-over-comb technique.

10. _____ cutting can be used to trim stray hairs from a hair design.

11. _____ tapering is useful for thinning out difficult areas of the hair caused by hollows, wrinkles, whorls, and creases in the scalp.

12. The method of marking the outer border of the haircut along the curved areas of the hairline at the bottom of the sideburn, in front of the ears, over the ears, and down the sides of the neck is called the _____.

13. Always protect the client's _____ when performing the _____ technique.

14. As a general rule, clipper cutting is followed up with _____ and _____ work to fine-tune the haircut.

15. Cutting the hair in the opposite direction from which it grows is called cutting _____.

16. Cutting _____ means cutting is performed in the same direction in which the hair grows.

17. When the hair is not cut with or against the grain, it is called cutting _____.

18. Cutting the hair in a _____ direction with the grain is advisable in whorl areas.

19. Arching can be performed with shears, _____, _____, or a razor.

20. Provide two reasons why is it important to consistently use the comb or hair pick while using the freehand clipper cutting technique. _____

_____

_____

21. A detachable clipper blade size 0000 cuts the hair close to _____ length.

22. A size 3½ clipper blade will leave the hair about _____ long.

23. Clipper attachment combs, or _____, are placed on top of a _____ and allow more hair length to remain while cutting.

24. Guards are generally _____ for state board practical examinations.

25. The clipper-over-comb cutting method is similar to the _____ technique.

26. Freehand clipper cutting, _____ work, and _____ work are frequently used to perform a single haircut.

27. For a gradual, even taper from shorter to longer hair, gradually tilt the clipper blade so that the clipper _____ of the bottom blade.

28. Match the following haircut descriptions or characteristics with the correct haircut style. Choices may be used more than once.

_____ crest area looks squared off

_____ even cut over the entire head

_____ very short on the sides and back areas

_____ also known as short pomp or brush cut

_____ three variations: short, medium, and long

_____ crown area is cut to between ¼" and ½" in length

_____ cut relatively high to the bottom of the crest area

_____ hair is uniformly cut close to the scalp

_____ crest has a slight curvature

_____ hair is cut with the grain to avoid gaps

a) flat top

b) crew cut

c) Quo Vadis

29. The primary _____ and _____ areas of haircut styles are classified as long cuts and trims, medium lengths, semi-short lengths, and short cuts.

30. A haircut in which the hair at the nape and sides is cut extremely close, blending to nothing at the hairline, is called a _____.

31. Gradually blending the fine clipper taper of a fade with the longer taper sections can be achieved by cutting with and _____ the grain as necessary.

32. Every effort should be made to make sure that the sideburns appear even in _____.

33. How should the length of the sideburns be checked? _____
_____

34. The _____ of the sideburns should be checked and trimmed so that they are complimentary to the facial shape and _____.

35. Razor cutting is especially suitable for _____, shortening, tapering, _____, or feathering specific areas.

36. Razor cutting can help make _____ hair textures more _____.

37. When razor cutting, the hair should always be in a clean and _____ condition.

38. The arm movement used in razor stroking and combing is done with _____ and the elbows are used as a hinge; _____ and arm movements can also be used.

39. In light taper-blending, the razor is held _____ against the surface of the hair with little pressure.

40. Heavier taper-blending is performed with the razor held up to _____ from the surface of the hair strand with a little more pressure.

41. The _____ of the razor and the amount of _____ determines the depth of the cut.

42. When the angle of the razor blade is almost _____, it is called terminal blending, hair-end tapering, or blunt cutting.

43. Razor stroking and combing are done in a _____ movement with one action following the other.

44. Which hair type requires more strokes and heavier tapering than other textures?
_____

45. Medium textured hair requires _____ razor strokes and _____ pressure than coarse, thick hair.

46. The razor can be used to blend the hair ends of _____ hair textures.

47. Gently stroking the razor to remove a thin sheet of hair from the section will taper the ends of the hair and _____.

48. When freehand slicing is used to cut the design line, it helps to create _____ perimeters.

49. Short, precise strokes with medium pressure applied to the hair surface are characteristics of the _____ technique.

50. When the comb and razor alternately follow each other through the hair, the technique is called _____ .

51. Sectioning the hair for a razor cut begins with combing the hair into the _____ effect.

52. List five razor cutting safety precautions in your own words.

1. _____

_____

2. _____

_____

3. _____

_____

4. _____

_____

5. _____

_____

53. Hair _____ is used to reduce the bulk or weight of the hair.

TOPIC 6: Shaving the Outline Areas

1. Haircutting finish work may include a _____ and an _____ .

2. Shaving the sides of the neck and across the nape with a razor is called a _____ .

3. An _____ consists of the sideburn areas, around the ears, and the nape area.

4. Many African American styles include the _____ in the outline shave.

5. Fill in the blanks where necessary to complete the preparation and performance steps of an outline shave.

1. Wash your hands.

2. Remove all cut hair from the client.

3. Loosen the chair cloth and remove the _____ .

4. Shake the chair cloth free of hair clippings.

5. Replace the chair cloth and a _____ around the client's neck, loosely.

6. Place a neckstrip or towel in the _____ of the chair cloth.

135

7. Apply shaving cream around the hairline.

8. Shave the right sideburn and side with the _____ stroke.

9. Shave the left sideburn with the _____ stroke.

10. Shave around the left ear using the _____ stroke.

11. Shave the left side of the neck using the _____ stroke.

12. Shave the nape area with a _____.

13. Shave the front hairline if requested by client; start in the _____ and work towards the corners using a _____ stroke to the right side and a _____ stroke to the left side. Shave along the _____ to the front corner of the sideburns.

TOPIC 7: Haircutting Procedures

1. Fingers-and-shear precision cut: Fill in the blanks as necessary to complete the primary preparation and performance steps of this technique.

   1. Wash your hands.

   2. Consult with the client.

   3. Drape for _____.

   4. _____ and towel dry hair.

   5. Drape for _____.

   6. Face client toward the _____ and _____ the chair.

   7. Cut top section from crown to front at _____ degrees using a traveling guide.

   8. Step to the side and hold top section at 90 degrees; establish _____ for _____ in _____; check top section at _____ from _____ to _____.

   9. Comb front down and establish front _____.

   10. Use front design line to cut from _____ to _____ in the _____.

   11. Establish _____ on both sides, then cut subsequent partings to _____.

   12. Take _____ partings on sides and hold at _____ degrees; cut from design line and blend to _____ and _____ sections.

   13. Establish _____ design line; connect nape design line to _____ design line; cut subsequent parting to perimeter guide.

   14. Use _____ partings held at 90 degrees in the back area to blend from the _____ to the _____ and _____ areas.

   15. Blend _____ to _____ section using vertical partings at 90 degrees.

136

16. Dry the hair and comb into place.

17. Clean up hairline with _____ or trimmer; perform a _____ or _____ shave as desired by client.

18. Re-comb hair and _____ according to client's wishes.

19. _____ or vacuum stray hairs.

2. What is the primary difference between the fingers-and-shear technique and the alternative fingers-and-shear technique? _____

_____

3. Shear-over-comb technique: Fill in the blanks as necessary to complete the primary preparation and performance steps of this technique.

1. Wash your hands.

2. _____

3. Drape for wet service.

4. _____ and towel dry hair. _____ hair if dry-cutting is preferred.

5. _____ for haircut.

6. Face client toward the mirror; lock the chair.

7. Comb the hair and use _____ technique to cut in the _____ area, trimming hair to the desired length and thickness up to the _____ .

8. Cut from the sideburn _____ into the side section on the right side.

9. Cut _____ and _____ the right ear.

10. Use a _____ comb position to blend hair _____ to the right corner of the nape.

11. Blend hair at the side of the neck into the _____ section.

12. Repeat on _____ side.

13. Blend hair from the _____ to the _____ .

14. Blend hair from the _____ through the right and left _____ areas into the _____ section.

15. Trim _____ to appropriate length.

16. Outline _____ , around the ear, and behind-the-ear areas with _____ , followed by the _____ .

17. Finish haircut with a _____ and/or outline _____ as desired by client.

18. Style the hair as desired.

19. Dust or vacuum stray hairs on the client's _____ and _____ .

137

4. Freehand and clipper-over-comb technique on straight hair: Fill in the blanks as necessary to complete the primary preparation and performance steps of this technique.

   1. Wash your hands.

   2. Consult with the client.

   3. Drape the model for a _____ service.

   4. _____ and towel dry hair. _____ hair if dry cutting is preferred.

   5. _____ for haircut.

   6. Face client toward the mirror and lock the chair.

   7. _____ the hair; start in the _____ area and _____ the first inch or so of hair.

   8. Use _____ cutting to the _____ and _____ areas.

   9. Establish the length of the _____ on the _____ side; begin clipper-over-comb cutting from the sideburn _____ into the _____ section.

   10. Continue technique _____ and in _____ of the right ear.

   11. Use a _____ comb position to _____ the hair behind the ear to the right _____ of the _____ along the _____ .

   12. Blend hair on the right side of the _____ into the back section.

   13. Repeat steps used on the right side on the left side.

   14. Blend hair from the _____ to the _____ .

   15. Blend hair from the _____ through the right and left _____ areas to meet the _____ sections.

   16. Trim _____ section using _____ method and cut to desired length; check _____ and fine-tune using fingers-and-shear method.

   17. Outline sideburns, _____ , and _____ areas with _____ and then trimmer.

   18. Complete _____ work by performing a neck shave after outlining the bottom of the sideburn and around-the-ear areas with a _____ .

   19. Style the hair as desired, then dust or vacuum stray hairs.

5. Freehand and clipper-over-comb technique on tightly curled hair: Fill in the blanks as necessary to complete the primary preparation and performance steps of this technique.

   1. Wash your hands.

   2. Consult with the client.

   3. Drape for wet service.

   4. Shampoo and towel dry hair. Blow-dry hair if dry cutting is preferred.

   5. Drape for haircut.

6. Face client toward the mirror and lock the chair.

7. Comb or _____ the hair out.

8. Start in _____ area; _____ taper or clipper-over-comb _____ the first inch or so of hair. If hair density allows, use _____ cutting to the occipital area. If the hair is _____, _____ clipper cut to the _____ area.

9. Cut in right side using freehand or clipper-over-comb technique to _____ and _____ from the _____ to the _____.

10. Continue technique _____ and in _____ of the right ear.

11. Use a diagonal comb position to blend the hair _____ to the hair at the _____ of the _____ along the _____; or, _____ the entire section.

12. Blend hair at the _____ of the neck into the _____ section.

13. Move to _____ side and begin _____ or _____ cutting from the sideburn hairline to the _____.

14. Continue technique _____ and in _____ of the _____ ear.

15. _____ the hair behind the ear to the hair at the left _____ of the _____ along the _____.

16. Blend hair at the side of the neck into the _____ section.

17. Establish guide in front _____ of _____ section; cut back to _____ area.

18. Blend _____ to _____ guide around the entire head.

19. Blend _____ area to _____; check the _____ to the _____ section.

20. Comb or pick hair out; fine-tune with _____.

21. Outline sideburns, around the ear, and back of the ear areas with _____ or _____.

22. Finish with neck and _____ shaving as requested by client.

23. Style the hair as desired, then dust or vacuum stray hairs from client's face and neck.

6. Razor cutting: Fill in the blanks as necessary to complete the primary preparation and performance steps of this technique.

1. Wash your hands.

2. Consult with the client.

3. Drape the model for wet service.

4. Shampoo and towel-dry hair.

5. Remove the waterproof cape and replace it with a neckstrip and haircutting cape.

6. Face model toward the mirror and lock the chair.

7. Section hair into _____ sections from _____ to _____, _____ to _____, and _____ to _____; subdivide the _____ section into _____ subsections.

8. Begin in the _____ section just below the _____; use razor _____ to taper _____ to the hairline; blend with previously cut hair.

9. Taper from _____ to _____ in the _____ section and the _____ section to blend with the _____ hair.

10. Repeat procedure from top _____ side toward _____ side.

11. Comb side hair downward and subdivide it into _____ vertical partings. Begin tapering about _____ " of an inch from the _____; taper downward through sections to _____. Comb hair _____ and taper to _____ with the back section; comb hair _____ and repeat blending to front design line.

12. Repeat procedure on _____ side of head.

13. Comb top hair _____; start tapering in top section; work toward the _____ on both sides of center, then taper the _____ section to blend all three sections; trim front section at _____ elevation using the _____ technique.

14. Comb to check for _____ and _____.

15. Perform neck _____ and/or _____ shave as desired by client.

16. Style the hair as desired by client; dust or vacuum stray hairs.

7. Fade cut: Fill in the blanks as necessary to complete the primary preparation and performance steps of this technique.

1. Wash your hands.

2. Conduct client consultation.

3. Drape the client for wet service.

4. Shampoo and towel dry hair.

5. Remove waterproof cape; replace with a _____ and haircutting cape.

6. Face client toward the mirror and lock the chair.

7. Set the clipper blade in the _____ position to achieve a close cut. Start at the _____ of the nape, cutting to the bottom of the _____. Cut right and left of center through the _____ section.

8. Move to either _____ of the client as preferred and cut from the hairline to the top, middle, or _____ of the crest area as desired by the client. Cut around the ear and into the previously cut _____ section, cutting up and/or _____ the growth pattern. Complete opposite side in the same manner.

9. With the back and sides completed, open the clipper blades _____ of the way for fine hair or almost _____ for thick hair. Cut a ¼" to ¾" thick section at the point where previous cutting was _____ at the crest. Continue cutting this section around the head.

10. Open the blades another _____ and repeat the procedure cutting another ¼" thick section above the one previously cut. Repeat as necessary.

11. Open the blades completely. Starting in the _____ area, blend the hair _____ the grain through the top and on a slight _____ into the shorter hair at the crest. Complete this step around the entire head.

12. Finish with the trimmer and/or outline shave to define the hairline.

13. Dust or vacuum stray hairs.

8. Head shaving: Fill in the blanks where necessary to complete the primary preparation and performance steps of this technique.

   1. _____ the scalp for any abrasions, primary or secondary lesions, or scalp disorders.

   2. Remove excess hair length with _____; use _____ clipper blade if available.

   3. Shampoo the remaining hair and _____ the scalp.

   4. Apply shaving cream or gel and lather; apply two or three _____ treatments.

   5. Use the _____ stroke to shave _____ the grain from the _____ to the _____ in the back section; follow the curve of the head, using _____ strokes with the first half of the blade from its _____ to _____.

   6. Move in _____ of client and tip his head _____ slightly; continue shaving from the _____ to the _____ hairline.

   7. When the top section is completed, work down the _____; hold the _____ out of the way and shave in front of and _____ the ears.

   8. Upon completion, check for any _____ areas.

   9. Remove remaining lather with a _____, apply _____ or _____, and follow with a _____ towel application for 2 to 3 minutes.

9. Haircutting finish work may include trimming excess hair from the _____, _____, and _____.

TOPIC 8: Men's Hairstyling

1. Hair styling is _____ _____.

2. Styling the hair may require the use of _____, blow-drying, or _____ the style into place.

3. Blow-drying offers options for _____ drying and _____ styling.

4. The nozzle is a directional feature that helps to _____ the air stream to a more _____ area.

5. A _____ attachment disperses the airflow to a larger area while allowing heat for drying purposes.

6. The methods used to style men's hair include natural drying, _____ styling, scrunch styling, _____, and blow-waving.

7. Freeform blow-drying can build _____ while allowing the hair to fall into the _____ lines of the cut.

8. Each section is dried in a definite direction with the aid of a comb or brush when using _____ blow-drying techniques. _____ is a form of stylized blow-drying.

9. _____ drying is used when the natural wave pattern of the hair is to be maintained.

10. To build volume, _____ the hair with a brush and _____ the section as the blow-dryer is directed at the _____ of the section. Follow through to the _____.

11. Styling techniques such as braids and locks are a form of _____ hair care.

12. _____ are one of the most popular braiding techniques chosen by men; fill in the blanks where necessary to complete the primary preparation and performance steps of this technique.

    1. Apply and massage essential _____ to the scalp.

    2. Determine the correct size and _____ of the cornrow _____; create two _____ partings to form a row for the base.

    3. Divide the parting into _____ strands; place fingers close to the base and cross the left strand under the center strand.

    4. Cross the right strand under the center strand.

    5. With each crossing-under, pick up hair from the base of the _____ and add it to the _____ strand before crossing it under the center strand.

    6. Braid subsequent panels in the same manner.

    7. Finish with oil sheen or an appropriate styling aid.

13. Locks are also known as _____.

14. Locks are created from _____-textured hair that is _____ together to form a single network of hair.

15. The process that occurs when coiled hair is allowed to develop in its natural state is called _____.

142

16. The term used to define hair that is intentionally guided through the natural process of locking is _____.

17. Some methods that are used to cultivate locks are _____, _____, and _____.

18. The most effective techniques for cultivating locks are _____ or _____ rolling.

19. What important considerations should be discussed with a client who is considering locks?

    a) _____

    _____

    b) _____

    _____

    c) _____

    _____

20. Fill in the blanks to complete the comb and rolling techniques used in locking the hair.

    a) The _____ technique is effective during the _____ stages of locking; it involves placing the comb at the _____ of the scalp and spiraling the hair into a curl with a _____ motion; with each revolution, the comb moves down along the _____ until it reaches the ends.

    b) Palm or finger rolling begins with _____ and conditioned hair; the hair is parted in horizontal rows from the _____ to the _____ hairline and divided into _____ subsections; gel is applied to the first subsection. Rolling begins at the _____ by using the index finger and thumb to pinch the hair near the scalp; then the strands are twisted in one full _____ revolution down the entire strand; after rolling, the hair is dried under a _____ on low heat; when the hair is completely dry, light oil is applied.

21. List nine safety precautions that should be used during haircutting and styling procedures:

    1. _____

    2. _____

    3. _____

    4. _____

    5. _____

    6. _____

    7. _____

    8. _____

    9. _____

Chapter 16: Men's Hair Replacement

Word Review

finasteride
flap surgery
full head bonding
hackling
hair replacement system

hair solution
hair transplantation
lace-front
minoxidil
root-turning

scalp reduction
styling or wig block
toupee

TOPIC 1: Introduction

1. Since ancient times, hairpieces and wigs have been worn to cover _____ areas, as part of ceremonial _____, or to conform to _____.

2. A small hairpiece or wig used to cover the top or crown of the head used to be called a _____.

3. Hair replacement options include drugs, hair replacement systems or solutions, surgical hair transplantation, and _____.

TOPIC 2: Hair Replacement Systems

1. The quality of a hair replacement varies with the kind of _____ used in its manufacture and the way in which it is _____.

2. The types of hair used in the construction of hair replacements are _____ hair, _____ hair, and _____ hair.

3. Some advantages of human hair include a more natural look and texture, durability, and the ability to tolerate _____ processes. Disadvantages include reactions to _____ changes and fading.

4. Special shampoos and conditioners are used on _____ hair systems.

5. _____ hair is used in the production of full wigs and some hair solutions.

6. Mixed-hair products are often used in the manufacture of _____ or fashion wigs.

7. Hair replacement systems are typically available with hard, _____, mesh, net, polyurethane, or _____ bases.

8. Materials used in base construction include silk, nylon, or plastic mesh; _____; thin _____ skin; or a combination of materials.

9. _____ refers to the way the hair is attached to the base of the hair solution.

10. Root-turning refers to sorting the hair strands so the cuticle points toward the hair ends in its _____ of growth.

11. Hair systems that are available from manufacturers and distributors in different sizes and colors are called _____ systems or _____ systems.

12. A custom hair replacement system requires a _____ or pattern and _____ matching.

13. Fill in the blanks to complete the questions a barber should ask a manufacturer before purchasing their hair replacement systems.

   a) What _____ materials are used in the construction of the hair solution?

   b) What _____ treatments have been applied?

   c) If human hair is used, is it graded in terms of _____ , elasticity, and porosity?

   d) Will the _____ stand behind their product?

   e) What is the _____ expectancy of the hair solution?

   f) Does the manufacturer have the ability to create _____ colors?

   g) Is _____ training offered about their products?

14. Most barbershops will already have many of the implements and supplies required for hair replacement services. Fill in the blanks with those items that may need to be obtained from a barber supply or hair replacement supply company.

   a) _____

   b) alcohol

   c) blow-dryer

   d) client record cards

   e) clippers

   f) comb

   g) _____

   h) envelopes

   i) grease pencil

   j) hair net

   k) haircutting shears

   l) _____

   m) _____

   n) plastic wrap or cellophane

   o) razor

   p) scissors (for cutting pattern)

   q) small brush

   r) _____

s) _____

t) thinning shears

u) _____

v) transparent tape

w) _____

15. The _____ is often the one to measure, fit, cut, and style the hair system once it has been received from the supplier.

16. When performing the _____, the hair should be lightly trimmed, leaving a low neckline and length close to the ears at the sides.

17. _____ from the preliminary cut are used as a texture and color guide.

18. The sizes of men's hair replacements are commonly measured in _____.

TOPIC 3: Templates and Molds

1. Fill in the blanks where necessary to complete the steps involved in measuring for stock and custom hair replacements.

   1. Place _____ fingers above the eyebrow, with the last finger resting on the bridge of the nose. Make a dot with a grease pencil on the forehead directly in line with the _____ to indicate where the hair system is to begin.

   2. Place the tape measure on the dot. Measure the length to where the _____ hair begins and mark the tape measure.

   3. Measure across the top, directly over the _____; measure across the _____ area if it is noticeably different from the front width.

   4. Assemble template-making materials.

   5. Place about 2 feet of _____ on top of the client's head and twist the sides until they conform to the contour of the head.

   6. Place four fingers above the eyebrows and make a dot on the _____ to indicate the _____ hairline. Place additional dots as follows:

      a) Two dots on each side where the _____ hairline will meet client's hairline

      b) Two dots in back of the head on each side of the _____ spot

      c) One dot at the center back edge of the bald spot to determine the _____ of the area to be covered

   7. Connect the dots with a pencil to outline the balding area.

   8. Place precut strips of tape across the bald area to _____ the pattern.

   9. Mark the front part of the pattern _____ and the back _____; remove and cut around the edge with scissors.

10. After cutting the outline, replace template over the balding area to make sure the bald area is _____ exactly.

11. Attach _____ of the client's hair to the pattern or client card for color matching by the manufacturer.

12. Create a client _____; send measurements and pattern to the manufacturer.

2. A _____ mold is a hard mold preferred by some manufacturers to create a more perfect fit.

3. When making a plaster mold, plaster _____ strips are applied over the plastic wrap instead of tape. Strips are applied from _____ to _____, then back to front and _____ the top.

4. Plaster molds need to cure for _____ hours before shipping to the manufacturer.

TOPIC 4: Customizing a Stock System

1. A plastic wrap and _____ template is used to customize a stock system.

2. The hair replacement system needs to be shampooed and _____ before cutting.

3. The hair replacement system is _____ or turned inside out on the canvas block.

4. The template is inverted and positioned _____ the hair system and secured with pins.

5. Using the template as a guide, a _____ is used to cut the base.

6. After the base has been cut, it must be checked for _____.

TOPIC 5: Applying and Removing Hair Replacement Systems

1. Before applying a replacement system, the bald area of the scalp needs to be cleaned with soap and water or _____.

2. Hair on the scalp should be removed wherever the _____ will be attached.

3. Both non-lace front and lace-front systems use _____ tape for attachment.

4. Tape should be applied to the _____ areas of the foundation only.

5. When applying either a non-lace front or lace-front system, the _____ measurement method above the _____ is used to locate the hairline for positioning of the system.

6. When removing a non-lace front replacement system, the tape needs to stay on the _____ so that it can be reactivated with _____.

7. Before removing a lace-front replacement system, the lace must be dampened with acetone or _____ to loosen it from the scalp.

8. _____ areas on a lace-front system with tape residue are cleaned gently with acetone or solvent.

9. _____ bonding is the process of attaching a hair replacement system to the head with an _____ bonding agent.

10. Copolymers are used for full head bonding and should be _____.

11. _____ coats of bonding adhesive should be applied to the client's scalp and _____ applied to the hair replacement system.

12. Because the hair replacement system will adhere to all parts of the scalp, the barber needs to stand behind the client and gradually _____ the system on from front to back without _____ the system or creating _____.

TOPIC 6: Cutting the Hair Replacement System

1. Removing excess length in the top section should be done at a _____ elevation.

2. Work in the top section is performed from the front of the _____ to the forehead using shears.

3. Side hair should be cut to blend with the _____ from the temple to the sideburn to the ear.

4. Hair on the sides is _____ gradually to the crest so the replacement system will be undetectable when blended with the client's natural hair.

5. In the back section, _____ are used to blend the ends of the hair replacement with the client's natural hair.

TOPIC 7: Other Hair Replacement Systems

1. _____ are lace fill-ins applied with spirit gum that may be used to cover scalp areas with a small degree of hair loss.

2. Facial hair solutions are attached with _____.

3. _____ wigs are usually made of synthetic fibers such as _____.

4. Full, ready-made wigs are usually constructed on a _____ made of lightweight elastic.

TOPIC 8: Cleaning and Styling Replacement Systems

1. Wigs should be cleaned with the manufacturer's recommended _____.

2. Hair replacement systems should be cleaned according to the _____ instructions.

3. Fill in the blanks where necessary to complete the steps for cleaning a human hair replacement system.

   a) Remove all the old tape and clean any reinforced areas by dabbing them lightly with _____.

    b) Put enough cleaner in a glass bowl so the system can be submerged. Invert the system with the _____ up and place into cleaning solution. Allow to soak for _____.

    c) _____ the system back and forth in the cleaner until all residue is removed from the hair and foundation.

    d) With a small brush, gently _____ of the hair system until adhesive is removed.

    e) If the solvent darkens, replace it with _____.

    f) Place the hair system on a towel with the inside _____. Gently _____ the cleaner with the towel.

    g) Hold replacement from the _____ section and comb gently.

    h) Fasten to a wig block and style or dry and _____ to client's scalp for styling.

4. Fill in the blanks where necessary to complete guidelines for basic hair replacement system care.

    a) Use the _____ tape, antiseptic, cleaner, and softeners.

    b) When the hair solution is not being worn, it should be placed on an appropriate _____.

    c) Some hair systems should be _____ for showering and swimming.

    d) Clean the hair solution after the _____ week of wear, and then every three to four weeks or as needed.

    e) Never _____ the hair solution.

    f) Always follow manufacturer's recommendations for _____ the hair replacement.

    g) Apply light hair dressings and sprays _____ and with even distribution.

    h) Set hair solutions with _____.

5. _____ treatments should be given as often as necessary to prevent dryness or brittleness of the hair.

6. Permanent haircoloring products can be used only on systems made of _____.

7. When permanent waving hair systems, the rod placement _____ rest on the scalp of the hair system.

8. Explain how rods are floated. _____
_____

9. The permanent waving process for a hair replacement system _____ require chemical neutralization; instead, the system is allowed to _____.

10. Fill in the blanks where necessary to complete general recommendations and reminders associated with hair replacement systems.

    a) Comb hair systems carefully to avoid _____, loss of hair, or damage.

    b) Use a _____ comb to avoid weakening or damaging the foundation.

c) Never rub or _____ cleaning fluids from the system. Let it dry naturally.

d) Be careful not to _____ too much hair when tapering and blending a system.

e) Take _____ measurements to assure a comfortable and secure fit.

f) _____ systems as often as necessary to prevent dryness, brittleness, or dullness of the hair.

g) If required, _____ systems before styling.

h) Brush and comb systems with a _____ movement.

i) To avoid damage to the foundation, never _____ or cold wave a system.

j) If _____ is necessary, it must be done with care.

11. List some marketing techniques discussed in the textbook, then provide an idea of your own.

a) _____

b) _____

c) _____

d) _____

e) _____

f) _____

g) _____

h) _____

TOPIC 9: Alternative Hair Replacement Methods

1. In addition to hair systems, two other options for hair replacement are _____ and _____.

2. _____ is a topical medication available for men and women.

3. Finasteride is an _____ medication prescribed to _____ only.

4. The process of removing hair from normal areas of the scalp and relocating them into bald areas under a local anesthetic is called _____.

5. Hair transplants are performed only by licensed _____ professionals.

6. The process by which the bald area is removed from the scalp and then surrounding scalp areas with hair growth are pulled together to fill in the spot is called _____.

7. _____ is the process of attaching a flap of hair-bearing skin to the bald area.

Chapter 17: Women's Haircutting and Styling

Word Review

base	hair molding	on-base
blow-dry styling	hair pressing	stem
blunt cut	hair wrapping	thermal styling
circle	half off-base	uniform layer cut
curl	long layer cut	
graduated cut	off-base	

TOPIC 1: Introduction

In certain shops, such as unisex salons, there is a fairly equal ratio of male to female clientele. In this environment, barbers must be proficient in cutting and styling women's hair as well as men's.

1. Many men's haircuts require very little _____ or _____ beyond combing the hair into place.

2. Most women's styles require some form of daily arranging with a _____, _____, or other tool.

3. One of the main differences between cutting women's hair and cutting men's hair is that men's cuts usually appear more _____ whereas women's cuts may be more _____ and soft looking.

4. Fill in the blanks to complete the following haircutting reminders:

    a) Start with clean and _____ hair.

    b) Pay attention to the _____ position.

    c) Pay attention to your _____.

    d) Pay attention to your _____ placement. Comb through and _____ the finger placement you will use before actually cutting the hair.

    e) Take consistent and clean _____ to produce more precise results.

    f) Keep the hair _____ when cutting.

    g) Work with _____ growth patterns.

    h) Use consistent _____.

    i) Always work with a _____ or _____. If you can't see the guide, _____!

    j) Use the _____ to check _____ and _____.

    k) Plan for the _____ factor that results when the hair dries or when cutting wavy and curly hair textures.

    l) Always check and _____ your work.

151

TOPIC 2: Basic Haircuts

1. The art of haircutting is made up of variations and combinations of four basic haircuts: the _____ , _____ , _____ , and _____ .

2. Different _____ and _____ are used to create different effects.

3. Identify each of the following characteristics as belonging to the blunt, graduated, uniform layered, or long layered cut.

    a) _____ has a wedge or stacked shape

    b) _____ hair looks like it is all the same length

    c) _____ hair is shorter in the top section, longer at the perimeter

    d) _____ all the hair strands are cut to the same length

    e) _____ also known as a one-length cut

    f) _____ created by cutting with tension at low to medium elevations

    g) _____ forms a weight line at the perimeter

    h) _____ hair is cut at 90 degrees from where it grows

    i) _____ hair is actually shorter underneath the top sections

    j) _____ achieved by using a 180-degree elevation

    k) _____ may be accomplished with horizontal or vertical partings

    l) _____ uses a stationary guide at the perimeter

    m) _____ commonly uses an elevation of 45 degrees

    n) _____ uses a stationary guide in the top section

    o) _____ has layers from 0 elevation to 45 degrees within the haircut

    p) _____ uses a traveling guide throughout the cut

    q) _____ cut at 0 elevation

    r) _____ consists of increased layering

4. Explain why less elevation might be used on curly hair textures.

    _____

    _____

5. Cutting the hair section in the trough of the wave may cause the hair ends to _____ from the head form.

6. Cutting just after the crest of the wave as it dips towards the trough may encourage the hair to fall _____ toward the _____ .

7. For curly hair textures, the amount of hair to be cut may have to be adjusted from one haircut to the next according to the _____ .

152

© 2011 Milady, a part of Cengage Learning. All Rights Reserved. May not be copied, scanned, or duplicated, in whole or in part, except for use as permitted in a license distributed with a certain product or service or otherwise on a password-protected website for classroom use.

8. Short natural cuts on extremely curly hair can be created using the _____ or _____ cutting techniques; the sides may be _____, _____, or _____ from the sides to the top section.

9. The decision to use clippers or shears depends on the _____ and _____ of the hair.

10. What is the rule for using fingers-and-shear cutting on extremely curly hair?

_____

_____

TOPIC 3: Other Techniques

1. Over-direction occurs when the hair is combed away from its _____ position.

2. The technique of shifting the hair into a different position to increase length in a design or to blend short and long lengths along a perimeter or interior section is called _____.

3. Razor cutting produces an _____ at the ends of the hair.

4. Razor cutting produces softer shapes with more _____ and visual _____ than shear-cut hair ends.

5. Texturizing techniques are used to remove excess bulk, add volume, create _____, or create _____ and _____ effects.

6. The most commonly used texturizing techniques are _____, _____, _____, _____, and _____.

7. When the tips of the shears are used on the hair ends at a steep angle in relation to the hair parting, the technique is called _____.

8. _____ is produced by positioning the shears at flatter angle to the ends of the hair; _____ is usually performed within the interior sections of a haircut.

9. The process of thinning the hair using a sliding shear movement with the blades kept partially opened is called _____.

10. _____ is performed with the shear blades open and cutting occurs at that part of the blade near the pivot.

11. A version of slicing that creates separation in the hair with an open and closing movement of the shears is called _____.

TOPIC 4: Hairstyling

1. The first step in the hairstyling process is the _____.

2. Consider the client's _____, hair texture, and lifestyle.

3. Hairstyling techniques include _____ hairstyling, _____ styling, _____ styling, and _____ styling.

4. The technique of wrapping hair around the head to create smooth styles is called
   _____.

5. _____ is the technique that involves combing the hair straight down and securing it with a wrapping strip while it dries.

6. Finger waving, pin curls, hair wrapping, hair molding, and roller sets are examples of wet setting or _____.

7. _____ is the process of shaping and directing the hair into an S-shaped pattern using the fingers, a comb, and setting lotion.

8. _____ are wound from the hair ends into a flattened curl spiral.

9. Roller sets are performed with tools called _____ that are used to set a pattern in the hair as a basis for a hairstyle.

10. Plastic rollers are used for most _____ roller sets; _____ rollers and _____ rollers are used on _____ hair only.

11. Hair _____ is a hairstyling method that uses the client's head as a form or tool.

12. Blow-dry styling may be used to prepare the hair for _____ curling techniques.

13. When the hair is allowed to dry naturally into a style with minimal manipulation, it is called
    _____.

14. Thermal styling includes thermal _____ and thermal hair straightening.

15. _____ tools are used to wave, curl, or straighten the hair in thermal styling processes.

16. Hair wrapping techniques may be used on wet or dry _____ and _____ hair textures to create a natural-looking _____ to the hairstyle.

17. Explain what to do when height or volume is desired at crown area in a hair wrap.

    _____

18. To increase volume in a blow-dry style, _____.

19. Thermal styling uses _____ to produce waving or straightening effects.

20. Thermal waving is achieved with conventional _____ or curling irons.

21. Thermal hair straightening is also known as _____.

22. Conventional Marcel irons and pressing combs require a _____ for heating.

23. The _____ size of the iron determines the size of the wave or curl.

24. The _____ of the hair from the scalp will determine where the curl sits in relation to its _____, and the amount of _____ achieved.

25. Use the terms *base, stem,* or *circle* to match the following definitions with the correct term. Choices may be used more than once.

a) _____ the hair between the scalp and the first arc of the barrel

b) _____ also known as the curl

c) _____ foundation on which the barrel or roller is placed

d) _____ part of the curl formed when hair is wrapped around the tool

e) _____ gives the hair direction and mobility

26. The three kinds of bases used in thermal and roller setting are: _____ , _____ , and _____ .

27. Use the terms *on-base, half-base,* and *off-base* to match the following characteristics with the correct term. Choices may be used more than once.

_____ placement that produces the least amount of volume

_____ also known as half off-base

_____ placement that sits directly on its base

_____ placement that sits completely off the base

_____ roller placement sits halfway on and halfway behind the base

_____ placement that produces a full volume curl

_____ achieved by slightly over-directing and rolling the hair beyond 90 degrees

_____ achieved by rolling the hair parting at 90 degrees

_____ achieved by holding and rolling the hair at 45 degrees from the base

28. Fill in the blanks to complete the steps for manipulating curling irons on a mannequin.

a) _____ the irons while opening and closing at regular intervals.

b) Rotate the irons _____ and upward.

c) _____ the hair by _____ the irons with a quick, clicking movement.

d) _____ the irons while opening and closing on the hair section.

e) Guide the hair section towards the _____ of the curl while rotating the irons.

f) Remove the curl from the irons by drawing the comb to the _____ and the curl to the _____ , using the comb to protect the scalp area.

29. Hair _____ temporarily straightens extremely _____ or hard to manage hair.

30. _____ pressing combs or electric _____ irons are used in hair pressing.

31. A _____ removes 50 to 60 percent of the curl.

32. A medium press removes _____ percent of the curl.

33. A _____ removes 100 percent of the curl.

34. Applying the pressing comb once to each side of the hair section is considered a
_____.

35. Applying the pressing comb twice to each side of the hair section is considered a
_____.

36. A _____, _____, or _____ is applied to shampooed
and dried hair prior to a pressing treatment to prevent the hair from _____ or
_____.

37. _____ thermal styling sprays also help to protect hair from heat damage.

38. Fill in the blanks to complete safety precautions associated with thermal styling tools.

    a) Use thermal irons only after receiving _____ on their use.

    b) Keep irons clean and _____.

    c) Always _____ the temperature of the iron before using on a client.

    d) Do not _____ irons.

    e) Handle and remove heated irons and stoves _____.

    f) Do not place heated stoves near a _____ as the heat can cause breakage.

    g) Place a _____ comb between the client's scalp and the iron. Never use a
_____ comb.

    h) Place heated stoves and irons in a _____ place to cool.

Date: _____

Rating: _____

Text Pages 566–611

Chapter 18: Chemical Texture Services

Word Review

acid-balanced waves
alkaline or cold waves
ammonium thioglycolate (ATG)
base control
base cream
base direction
base relaxers
base sections
basic perm wrap
bookend wrap
chemical blow-out

chemical hair relaxing
chemical texture services
croquignole rodding
disulfide bonds
end wraps
endothermic waves
exothermic waves
glyceryl monothioglycolate
  (GMTG)
hydroxide relaxers
lanthionization

lotion wrap
neutralization
no-base relaxers
permanent waving
prewrap solution
reformation curl
texturize
thio relaxer
true acid waves

TOPIC 1: Introduction

Chemical texture services such as permanent waving, reformation curls, and relaxers create chemical changes that permanently alter the natural wave pattern of the existing hair growth.

1. Chemical services can be used to _____ straight hair, _____ in curly hair types, or _____ hair that is too curly.

2. _____ applications are required to maintain altered textures when new growth occurs.

3. The process that chemically restructures straight or wavy hair into a different wave formation is called _____.

4. A _____ is a process used to restructure very curly hair into a larger curl pattern.

5. _____ is the process used to rearrange the structure of hair that is overly curly into a straighter hair form.

TOPIC 2: The Nature of Chemical Texture Services

1. Chemical texture services create _____ changes in the structure and appearance of the hair.

2. The two layers of the hair most affected by chemical texture services are the _____ and _____.

3. The degree to which hair is resistant to chemical changes depends on the strength of the _____.

4. _____ solutions and substances used in chemical texture services _____ and _____ the _____, allowing for penetration into the _____.

5. The _____ gives the hair its strength, flexibility, elasticity, and shape; _____ bonds in the cortex are _____ or _____ with chemical texture services.

6. Cysteine is an amino acid obtained by the _____ of cystine.

7. Reduction facilitates the chemical _____ of the inner structure of the hair as it assumes a new shape and form; the hair must then be _____ to ensure permanent reformation of the bonds in the cortical layer.

8. Chemical texture services involve _____ and _____ actions on the hair.

9. The three physical actions involved in permanent waving are _____, _____, and _____; the chemical actions are _____ and _____.

10. The three physical actions involved in the reformation curl process are _____, _____, and _____; the chemical actions are facilitated by the _____, _____ or _____, and _____.

11. The difference between the waving lotion and the rearranger is one of _____.

12. The five physical actions involved in chemical hair relaxing are _____ or _____, _____, _____, and _____.

13. The primary _____ action that occurs in hair relaxing is the result of the relaxer product used to straighten the hair.

14. Hydroxide relaxing products are neutralized through the _____ actions of shampooing and rinsing. Why? _____
_____

15. Thio relaxing products require the use of a _____ to chemically _____ the hair.

16. Hydroxide relaxers and thio relaxers _____ compatible.

17. The permanent breakage of disulfide bonds with a chemical relaxer is known as _____.

18. Hydroxide relaxers are strong _____ that can have a pH as high as _____.

TOPIC 3: The Client Consultation

1. The barber should ask the client _____ to determine the client's desires and past experience with chemical texture services.

158

2. List four topics that may be discussed during the client consultation.

a) _____

b) _____

c) _____

d) _____

_____

3. Client information and service outcomes should be recorded on a _____ .

4. A _____ and _____ analysis must be performed before proceeding with any chemical texture service; the analysis is used to determine the advisability of the service and the _____ that should be used in the procedure.

5. Do not proceed with a chemical service if _____ or signs of scalp _____ are present.

6. A hair analysis includes determining the hair's _____, _____, _____, _____, _____, and _____ .

7. The _____ level of the hair helps to determine the most appropriate _____ of chemical product to use.

8. Identify the following characteristics as describing *resistant*, *normal*, or *porous* hair.

a) _____ has a raised cuticle layer

b) _____ neither resistant nor overly porous

c) _____ tight, compact cuticle layer

d) _____ requires a more alkaline solution

e) _____ services usually process as expected

f) _____ absorbs solutions easily

g) _____ inhibits penetration of chemical solutions

h) _____ requires a less alkaline solution

9. Explain how to perform a porosity test.

_____

_____

_____

10. How can you tell if the hair is porous?

_____

11. If the fingers slide easily and no ruffles are formed, the hair is probably _____ .

12. Hair texture helps to determine the _____ .

13. _____ hair usually requires processing than medium or fine hair.

14. Hair _____ indicates the _____ of the cross-bonds in the hair.

15. Explain how to perform an elasticity test.

    _____

    _____

    _____

16. Signs of _____ elasticity include limpness, sponginess, and hair that tangles easily.

17. Hair _____ helps to determine the number of blockings or _____ that will best facilitate the chemical service and how much _____ will be needed.

18. Hair _____ may determine the _____ to use or how much _____ will be required for the service.

19. The _____ pattern of the hair helps to determine wrapping patterns and rod placement in _____ and _____ and the direction of _____ and _____ in chemical hair relaxing.

TOPIC 4: Permanent Waving

1. Permanent waves are performed on hair that has been freshly _____ and is in a _____ condition.

2. _____ moisture content should be maintained throughout the hair while rodding the perm.

3. List the factors that influence the size and shape of the curl in a permanent wave.

    a) _____

    b) _____

    c) _____

    d) _____

4. The size or _____ of the rod determines the size of the curl.

5. The most commonly used rods are _____ and _____ rods.

6. Review the following characteristics of rods and identify the style as concave or straight.

    a) _____ rods with a larger diameter at both ends

    b) _____ the most commonly used perm rods

    c) _____ rods with a smaller diameter in the center

    d) _____ rods with a uniform circumference

    e) _____ rods that produce tighter curl in the center

    f) _____ rods used for definite wave pattern, close to the head

    g) _____ rods with a uniform diameter along the length

7. Absorbent papers used to control the ends of the hair when winding the hair on perm rods are called _____ or _____ .

8. A _____ is a flaw in the wrapping procedure that bends the tip of the hair opposite to the direction of the rest of the curl.

9. The _____ wrap uses one paper folded in half over the hair ends; the _____ or _____ wrap uses one paper placed over the top of the hair parting; and the _____ wrap uses two end papers, one under and one over the hair parting.

10. Perm wraps begin with sectioning the hair into _____ ; each panel is divided into subsections called _____ .

11. Base sections should measure _____ the same length and width of the rod.

12. What will be the result if the rod is shorter than the blocking or subsection?

    _____

    _____

13. Identify the characteristics of the hair that help to determine the following: how the hair should be sectioned and subsectioned, which rods to use, and where the application of waving solution should begin. _____

14. What is base control? How is it determined?

    _____

    _____

15. Use the terms *on-base*, *half-base*, and *off-base* to match the following characteristics with the correct term. Choices may be used more than once.

    a) _____ placement that produces the least amount of volume

    b) _____ also known as half off-base

    c) _____ placement that sits directly on its base

    d) _____ placement that sits completely off the base

    e) _____ placement sits halfway on and halfway behind the base

    f) _____ placement that produces a full-volume curl

    g) _____ achieved by over-directing the hair beyond 90 degrees

    h) _____ achieved by rolling the hair parting at 90 degrees

    i) _____ achieved by holding the hair at 45 degrees from the base

16. What does base direction refer to? _____

    _____

17. What three partings and positions might be used for rod placement?

    _____

18. In the _____ rodding technique, the hair is wound from the ends to the scalp.

161

19. _____ rodding is accomplished by positioning the rod vertically and rodding from the ends to the scalp, or from the scalp to the ends.

20. The two types of wrapping methods used in permanent waving are the _____ wrap and the _____ wrap.

21. What is the difference between a water wrap and a lotion wrap?

    _____

    _____

22. What is the purpose of a lotion wrap? With what type of waving lotion is it used?

    _____

23. Review the following characteristics of permanent waves, then match to the correct type. Choices may be used more than once.

    _____ main active ingredient is ATG

    _____ usual pH between 7.8 and 8.2

    _____ most require heat from a hair-dryer

    _____ contain sulfates, sulfites, or bisulfites

    _____ used on resistant hair types

    _____ usual pH range of 4.5 to 7.0

    _____ contains an activator with GMTG

    _____ usually marketed as body waves

    _____ strong curl patterns; faster processing time

    _____ produces a softer, natural looking curl

    _____ maintains a constant pH level

    _____ releases heat when mixed

    _____ used on delicate hair types

    _____ usual range of 9.0 to 9.6

    _____ contains ATG and GMTG

    _____ evaporates slowly

    _____ may be water or lotion wrapped

    _____ primary reducing agent is GMTG

    _____ produces firmer curls than true-acid waves

    _____ do not produce a firm curl

    _____ has an activator with hydrogen peroxide

    _____ considered to be endothermic perms

    _____ uses alkanolamines

    _____ primary reducing agent is cysteamine or mercaptamine

    a) true-acid perms

    b) alkaline perms

    c) exothermic waves

    d) acid-balanced waves

    e) thio-free waves

    f) low-pH waves

    g) ammonia-free waves

24. Name three strengths of permanent waving products manufacturers usually produce and the types of hair they are intended for.

a) _____

b) _____

c) _____

25. What is a pre-wrap and what does it do?

_____

_____

_____

26. Resistant hair types usually require an _____ wave.

27. Most normal hair types can be permed with _____ or _____ perms.

28. _____ or _____ perms are the usual choice for tinted, highlighted, or delicate hair types.

29. The amount of processing time depends on the _____
and the _____ .

30. Most processing takes place within the first _____ to _____ minutes.

31. The wave has reached its peak when it forms a firm letter _____ shape.

32. Frizziness is an indication of _____-processing.

33. A weak wave formation is an indication of _____-processing.

34. What is the purpose of a test curl? _____

_____

35. What important aspects of a permanent wave service can be observed from a test curl?

a) _____

b) _____

c) _____

d) _____

e) _____

36. What are neutralizers? _____

_____

37. The most common neutralizer is _____ .

38. Name two other types of neutralizers. _____

39. What are two important functions of a neutralizer? _____

_____

_____

40. What important step should be included in the neutralization process after the waving lotion has been rinsed from the hair? Why?

_____

_____

_____

41. A mild _____ shampoo and a _____ conditioner should be recommended for permed hair.

42. The five common wrapping patterns used in permanent waving are the _____, _____, _____, _____, and _____ wraps.

43. One of the best wrapping patterns for men's styles is the _____ perm wrap.

44. When only a portion of the hair is permed, it is called a _____.

45. _____ treatments should be given to dry, damaged hair prior to a permanent wave service.

46. Fill in the blanks to complete the following safety precautions associated with permanent waving.

   a) Always protect clients clothing with a _____ drape.

   b) Use two towels; one _____ the drape and one over the drape.

   c) Always _____ the client's scalp before a perm service; _____ proceed if abrasions are present.

   d) Do not proceed with the perm if the client has ever experienced a/an _____ reaction to the products.

   e) Do not perm excessively _____ hair or hair that has been treated with _____ relaxers.

   f) Always apply a _____ barrier around the client's hairline before applying the cotton coil and waving solution.

   g) Immediately replace _____ cotton coils or towels.

   h) Always protect the client's _____ with a _____ when applying waving and neutralizing solutions.

   i) Always follow the _____ directions.

   j) Do not _____ or _____ to solutions unless specified by the manufacturer.

   k) Wear _____ when applying solutions.

   l) Do not save _____ or unused products.

   m) Unless otherwise specified in the _____, apply solutions liberally to the top and underside of each rod.

   n) Start applications at the crown or top and progress systematically _____ each section.

   o) Follow the same _____ for the neutralizer as used with the waving solution.

164

47. If it becomes necessary to re-saturate the rods during processing, watch the _____ development closely.

48. In your own words, list the preparation and procedural steps for a permanent wave service. Some of the steps have been provided for you.

    1. Wash your hands.

    2. _____

    3. _____

    4. Select and arrange required materials.

    5. Drape client for a shampoo.

    6. _____

    7. Perform preliminary test curl.

    8. Cut hair (optional).

    9. _____

    10. Rod the hair.

    11. _____

    12. Give client a towel to protect the eyes.

    13. _____

    14. Check curl formation according to manufacturer's directions.

    15. Process hair for required time.

    16. Apply fresh cotton strip.

    17. _____

    18. _____

    19. _____

    20. Remove rods carefully.

    21. Apply remaining neutralizer and work through the hair.

    22. _____

    23. Towel dry and style.

TOPIC 5: Reformation Curls

    1. A reformation curl is also known as a _____ permanent.

    2. Soft curl permanents are used to _____ very curly hair into looser and larger curls.

    3. Reformation curls use a thio _____ , thio _____ , and a _____ .

    4. Activators and moisturizers are _____ .

165

5. The thio relaxer used in a reformation curl service is commonly called the _____.

6. The thio waving solution is called the _____.

7. The neutralizer is an _____.

8. The _____ wrap method is used to rod a reformation curl service.

9. In your own words, list the preparation and procedural steps for a reformation curl service. Some of the steps have been provided for you.

    1. _____

    2. Conduct client consultation.

    3. _____

    4. Select and arrange required materials.

    5. _____

    6. Part the hair into four sections.

    7. _____

    8. Wear gloves; apply rearranger to top and underside of the parting.

    9. _____

    10. Process according to directions and rinse thoroughly.

    11. Part hair into panels for rodding.

    12. _____

    13. Continue booster application and rodding in each panel.

    14. _____
    _____

    15. Apply plastic cap if recommended.

    16. Replace saturated cotton and towels.

    17. Process according to directions.

    18. _____

    19. Rinse thoroughly; towel blot each rod.

    20. _____

    21. Remove rods and distribute the remaining neutralizer; rinse thoroughly.

    22. Shampoo and condition according to manufacturer's directions.

    23. Style the hair as desired.

TOPIC 6: Chemical Hair Relaxing

1. Chemical hair relaxing is the process of _____ rearranging the basic structure of extremely _____ hair into a _____ form.

2. The basic products used in the chemical hair relaxing process are _____ or _____, _____ or _____ shampoos, _____, and _____.

3. The two most common types of relaxers are _____ and _____ relaxers.

4. The type of relaxer that may require pre-service shampooing is the _____ relaxer.

5. Thio relaxers require the application of a _____ neutralizing solution.

6. Hydroxide relaxers are neutralized through the physical actions of _____ and _____ with an _____ or neutralizing shampoo product.

7. The ATG used in chemical relaxers is _____ than the ATG used in permanent waving.

8. Thio relaxers usually have a pH above _____.

9. Sodium hydroxide relaxers are known as _____ relaxers.

10. Sodium hydroxide relaxers can have a pH range of _____ to over _____.

11. _____ and _____ hydroxide relaxers are often sold as "no mix, no lye" relaxers.

12. Guanidine hydroxide relaxers are usually advertised as _____ relaxers.

13. No-lye relaxers contain a relaxer cream and an _____ that are mixed immediately prior to use and are recommended for _____ scalps.

14. _____ hydroxide relaxers may be mistakenly referred to as "no-lye" relaxers.

15. Calcium hydroxide relaxers require the addition of an activator; however, the strength of the relaxer is determined by the _____ used in the mixture.

16. Hydroxide relaxers are usually sold in _____ and _____ formulas.

17. _____ relaxers require the application of a _____ to scalp prior to relaxer application; _____ relaxers contain a base cream and do not require the application of a separate protective base.

18. Most chemical relaxers are available in _____, _____, and _____ strengths.

19. Relaxing products can be used to _____ extremely curly hair or to perform a _____ service.

20. When using sodium hydroxide for a chemical blow-out service, _____ is very important and the chemical should not be kept on the hair for more than _____ of the recommended processing time.

21. Fill in the blanks where necessary to complete the safety precautions associated with performing chemical hair relaxing services.

    1. Always protect clients' clothing with a waterproof drape.

    2. Use two towels; one under the drape and one _____ the drape.

    3. Always examine the client's scalp before a relaxer service. Do not proceed if abrasions are present.

    4. _____ if the client has ever experienced an allergic reaction to the products.

    5. Do not relax excessively _____ hair.

    6. Do not use a _____ relaxer on hair that has been treated with a hydroxide relaxer.

    7. Always apply a protective _____ barrier around the client's hairline before applying the relaxer.

    8. Base the _____ with a protective cream as directed by the product manufacturer.

    9. Always be careful of the client's eyes when applying relaxers and neutralizing solutions. In case of accidental exposure, rinse thoroughly with _____ water.

    10. Always follow the manufacturer's directions.

    11. Do not _____ or add anything to relaxer creams unless specified in the manufacturer's directions.

    12. Wear _____ when applying relaxers.

    13. Do not save _____ or _____ products.

    14. Apply relaxer cream to the most _____ area first.

    15. Follow the same pattern for smoothing the relaxer as was used during the application process.

22. Depending on the manufacturer's directions, shampooing before a thio relaxer is

    _____.

23. In your own words, list the preparation and procedural steps for a virgin thio or hydroxide relaxer application. Some of the steps have been provided for you.

    1. Wash your hands.

    2. _____

    3. Perform hair and scalp analysis.

    4. _____ and arrange required materials.

    5. Drape client for a chemical service. A _____ is optional for the thio relaxer service.

    6. Section the hair into four sections.

    7. _____

    8. Base the scalp.

9. Wear gloves and apply the relaxer _____ from the scalp on both sides of the parting.

10. _____

11. Process according to manufacturer's directions; _____
_____ during the last few minutes of processing.

12. Carefully comb and smooth all sections.

13. _____

14. Thio relaxer neutralization: Apply normalizing or _____; comb through to hair ends; process and _____ thoroughly; follow manufacturer's directions for _____ and _____.

15. _____ relaxer neutralization: Shampoo at least _____ times with an acid-balanced _____ shampoo; rinse thoroughly and condition according to manufacturer's directions.

16. Style as desired.

24. When performing a relaxer retouch application, the relaxer product is applied _____ from the scalp on the top and underside of the _____.

25. Care must be taken when applying relaxer product on new growth to not _____ the relaxer onto previously relaxed hair.

Chapter 19: Haircoloring and Lightening

Word Review

activator	hair lightening	primary colors
aniline derivatives	highlighting	progressive colors
base color	hue	retouch application
cap technique	laws of color	secondary colors
color fillers	level	semipermanent color
complementary color	level system	single-process haircoloring
contributing pigment	lightener	soap cap
demipermanent color	line of demarcation	strand test
developer	lowlighting	temporary colors
double-process haircoloring	off-the-scalp lighteners	tone
dye remover	on-the-scalp lighteners	toners
filler	patch test	virgin application
foil technique	permanent haircolor	volume
freeform technique	pre-lightening	
haircoloring	pre-softening	

TOPIC 1: Introduction

Men and women have altered their hair color for thousands of years. Early man considered colors to be symbols of power and mysticism.

1. Hair _____ is the science and art of changing the color of the hair.

2. Hair _____ is the partial or total removal of _____ pigment or _____ color from the hair.

3. Clients may request color changes if they want a fashion change, are prematurely _____, or wish to have decorative effects such as _____ or _____.

4. A skilled haircolorist is proficient in adding _____ pigment to _____, previously _____, or _____ hair and understands the process of _____ natural pigment through _____ agents.

TOPIC 2: Characteristics and Structure of Hair

1. Hair structure affects the _____ and outcome of the haircolor service.

2. Characteristics of the hair's structure should be used when determining haircoloring options and product selection. These characteristics include the strength of the _____, _____, _____, _____, _____, and natural _____.

3. _____ is distributed differently within different hair textures. _____ -textured hair has an average response time to color products; _____ hair may take longer to process.

4. To assure proper coverage of haircoloring or lightening products, the _____ of the hair should be considered.

5. The porosity level of the hair influences its ability to _____ .

6. Use the terms *porous*, *low porosity*, *average porosity*, or *high porosity* to identify each characteristic with the correct porosity level.

   a) _____ color may fade sooner than other porosity levels

   b) _____ permits darker saturation of color

   c) _____ hair tends to process in an average amount of time

   d) _____ hair that is resistant to moisture

   e) _____ may require a longer processing time

   f) _____ hair that may take color quickly

   g) _____ hair with a tight cuticle

   h) _____ hair with a lifted cuticle

   i) _____ hair with a slightly raised cuticle

   j) _____ accepts haircolor products faster

   k) _____ hair that may not hold color

7. _____ gives black and brown color to hair; _____ is the _____ found in yellowish-blonde, ginger, and red tones.

8. Three factors that determine all natural colors are the _____ of the hair, the total _____ and _____ of pigment granules, and the _____ of eumelanin to pheomelanin.

9. _____ hair is the color of keratin without melanin.

10. The pigment that lies under the natural hair color is called _____ .

11. The amount of gray in an individual's hair is measured in _____ . Identify the percentage of gray indicated by the following conditions.

   a) more gray than pigmented: _____

   b) more pigmented than gray hair: _____

   c) virtually no pigmented hair: _____

   d) even mixture of gray and pigmented hair: _____

TOPIC 3: Color Theory

1. Color is a form of visible _____ .

2. The laws of color regulate the mixing of _____ and _____ to make other colors.

3. Match with the correct term or word with its description. Choices may be used more than once.

   _____ yellow and this create green

   _____ yellow, red, and blue

   _____ colors with a predominance of blue

   _____ colors that are predominantly red

   _____ the darkest and only cool primary color

   _____ blue and this create violet

   _____ primary that brightens other colors

   _____ red-orange and yellow-orange

   _____ makes blue-based colors appear lighter

   _____ red and green

   _____ the lightest primary color

   _____ the medium primary color

   _____ violet and yellow

   _____ red and this create orange

   _____ yellow-green and blue-green

   _____ creates depth or darkness to a color

   _____ orange and blue

   _____ blue-violet and red-violet

   _____ composed of a primary and a secondary color

   _____ created by mixing equal amounts of two primary colors

   _____ colors located across from each other on the color wheel

   _____ colors that cannot be created by combining other colors

   a) primary colors

   b) cool-toned colors

   c) blue

   d) warm-toned colors

   e) red

   f) yellow

   g) secondary colors

   h) tertiary colors

   i) complementary colors

4. When mixed in equal amounts, complimentary colors _____ each other.

5. The basic name of a color is called its _____ or _____ .

6. Tone also describes the _____ or _____ of a color.

7. Warm colors are also known as _____ colors.

8. Cool colors are also known as _____ or _____ colors.

172

9. In haircoloring, the lightness or darkness of a color is called the _____ of the color.

10. In haircoloring, the _____ is used to analyze the lightness or darkness of a hair color.

11. Hair colors are arranged on a scale of _____; black is number _____; _____ is lightest blond.

12. The degree of concentration or amount of pigment in the color is called _____ or _____.

13. A _____ color is the predominant tone of a color.

14. What is the first step in performing a haircolor service and how is it accomplished?

_____

_____

15. Haircoloring results are based on the combination of the _____ color and the _____ color that is added to it.

TOPIC 4: Haircoloring Products

1. The classifications of haircoloring products indicate color-fastness, which is

_____.

2. Haircoloring products are categorized as _____ or _____. The four classifications of haircoloring products are _____, _____, _____, and _____.

3. Review the following characteristics of haircoloring products and identify each with the correct type: *temporary*, *semipermanent*, *demipermanent*, or *permanent* color products.

   a) _____ colors with the greatest pigment molecular weight

   b) _____ color rinses

   c) _____ will last from six to eight shampoos

   d) _____ deposits color without lifting

   e) _____ usually contains ammonia, oxidative tints, and peroxide

   f) _____ regarded as the best products for covering gray

   g) _____ self-penetrating

   h) _____ must be mixed with a low-volume developer

   i) _____ can lighten and deposit color in one process

   j) _____ coats the outside of the hair strand

   k) _____ haircolor sprays

   l) _____ considered a penetrating tint

m) _____ chemical composition is acidic

n) _____ does not develop color

o) _____ may serve as non-peroxide toner on pre-lightened hair

p) _____ mixed with a 20-developer

q) _____ tends to fade with each shampoo

r) _____ referred to as semipermanent by some manufacturers

s) _____ requires retouch applications

t) _____ ranges between 9.0 and 10.5 on the pH scale

u) _____ has a pH range of 2.0 to 4.5

v) _____ requires a patch test

w) _____ does not penetrate the cuticle layer

x) _____ color-enhancing shampoo

y) _____ chemical composition is mildly alkaline

z) _____ considered a type of oxidation color

aa) _____ also known as direct dyes

bb) _____ haircolor product that falls within the 7.0 to 9.0 pH range

cc) _____ darkens the natural hair color when applied

dd) _____ amount of lift is controlled by peroxide concentration

ee) _____ lasts from shampoo to shampoo

ff) _____ remains in the hair shaft

gg) _____ capable of lifting one or two levels

hh) _____ patch test is not required

ii) _____ partially penetrates into the cortex

jj) _____ also known as no-lift, deposit-only haircolor

4. Temporary and true semipermanent haircolor are considered _____ color products.

5. Demipermanent and permanent haircolor are considered _____ color products; however, demipermanent haircolor is also a no-lift, _____ color product.

6. Permanent haircolor is considered a _____ tint because it is mixed with an _____ that allows penetration into the cortex. This action is facilitated by _____ in the color product.

7. Toners are a type of _____ color and contain aniline derivatives.

8. Haircolor products made from various plants are called _____.

174

9. _____ or _____ or dyes are advertised as color restorers or _____ colors and _____ professional coloring products.

10. _____ are metallic or mineral dyes combined with a vegetable tint and are not used professionally.

11. A _____ is an oxidizing agent used for the development of color; most developers range between _____ and _____ on the pH scale.

12. The primary oxidizing agent used in haircoloring is _____ .

13. Diffused melanin is called _____ .

14. The term _____ is used to denote the different strengths of hydrogen peroxide; the higher the volume, the _____ the lifting action.

15. Permanent haircolor products use _____ , _____ , _____ , or _____ -volume hydrogen peroxide for proper color development; the majority of permanent coloring products use _____ -volume hydrogen peroxide.

16. Hydrogen peroxide is also known as _____ , _____ , _____ , or _____ .

17. Hydrogen peroxide is available in _____ , _____ , or _____ form.

18. Fill in the blanks to complete hydrogen peroxide safety precautions.

    1. Use clean implements when _____ , using, and storing hydrogen peroxide.

    2. Never measure the needed amount by pouring it into the _____ of another product.

    3. Do not allow hydrogen peroxide formulations to come in contact with _____ .

    4. Avoid _____ caused by mixing hydrogen peroxide and haircolor products.

    5. 20-volume or greater hydrogen peroxide can cause skin irritations, _____ , and hair damage.

    6. Dispose of plastic bottles of hydrogen peroxide that develop a _____ .

19. What is an activator? _____

20. What is the purpose of an activator? _____

21. Chemical compounds that lighten hair by _____ , _____ , and _____ the natural hair pigment are called lighteners.

22. When mixed for use, lighteners have a pH around _____ on the pH scale.

23. Hair can go through up to _____ stages of lightening.

24. Hair lighteners are used to create _____ shades not possible with permanent haircolor.

25. Lighteners are available in three forms: _____, _____, and _____; oil and cream lighteners are considered _____ lighteners; powder lighteners are _____ lighteners.

26. Oil lighteners are mixtures of hydrogen peroxide with _____ oil and are the _____ form of lightener.

27. Color oil lighteners add _____ color, highlight the hair as they lighten, and contain _____ colors.

28. _____ lighteners are the most popular type of on-the-scalp lightener.

29. _____ lighteners work quickly and do not contain conditioning agents.

30. Lighteners should not be used when the scalp shows sensitivity or _____.

31. _____ pigment that remains in the hair after lightening contributes to the _____ color that is added.

32. Use Figure 19-14 in your text to match the following color levels to the correct contributing pigment.

_____ black	a) red-orange
_____ very dark brown	b) pale yellow
_____ dark brown	c) blue
_____ medium brown	d) red
_____ light brown	e) blue-violet
_____ dark blond	f) yellow
_____ medium blond	g) red-violet
_____ light blond	h) yellow-orange
_____ very light blond	i) violet
_____ lightest blond	j) orange

33. _____ are applied to pre-lightened hair to achieve the desired color or shade in the hair.

34. Toners differ from tints in the degree of color _____ and require a _____ test.

35. Over-lightened hair will grab the _____ color of the toner.

36. _____ removers are also known as color or tint removers.

37. _____ have the ability to create a color base and equalize excessive porosity and are available in _____ , _____ , and _____ bases.

38. _____ are commercially prepared solutions that remove most tint stains from the skin.

TOPIC 5: Haircoloring Procedures Terminology

1. A patch test is also known as a _____ test; this test must be given _____ hours prior to the application of an aniline derivative tint or toner.

2. Fill in the blanks to complete the steps for performing a patch test.

    1. Select _____ area.

    2. _____ test area with mild soap and water.

    3. Dry test area by _____ with cotton or towel.

    4. Prepare test _____ according to manufacturer's directions.

    5. Apply solution to test area with _____ applicator.

    6. Leave test area uncovered and undisturbed for _____ .

    7. Examine test area for negative or positive _____ .

    8. Record results on client's _____ .

3. A _____ test will show no signs of inflammation and indicates the color may be applied safely.

4. A _____ test produces redness, swelling, burning, itching, blisters, or eruptions.

5. A _____ test helps to determine how the hair will react to the haircolor product, how long it will take to process, and what it will look like.

6. Fill in the blanks to complete the steps for a strand test procedure.

    1. Part off a _____ square parting of hair.

    2. Place the parting over a piece of _____ or plastic wrap; mix haircoloring product and apply to the hair strand.

    3. Check development time every _____ minutes until desired color is achieved; note time on record card.

    4. When color has developed, remove foil; place towel under the section; _____ , add shampoo, and massage through the strand; rinse, towel dry strand, and observe _____ .

    5. Adjust _____ , product formulation, or application as necessary.

7. What is a soap cap and what is it used for? _____
_____
_____

8. The term used to describe the process of returning a client to their natural shade is a
_____.

9. A client _____ should be completed for each client and contain all information pertaining to the haircoloring service.

10. A _____ is a form that should be used when the client's hair is in a questionable condition to withstand chemical processes and treatments.

11. Fill in the blanks to complete the steps for performing a haircoloring service client consultation.

   1. _____ the client.

   2. Have _____ fill out contact information on client record card.

   3. Perform _____ analysis, log results on record card, and determine _____ color level.

   4. Ask _____ questions about the desired end result.

   5. Show _____ of appropriate colors; decide color with the client.

   6. Review the procedure, application technique, _____, and cost with the client.

   7. Gain approval and perform _____ and _____ tests.

   8. Record end _____ on client record card.

TOPIC 6: Haircolor Application Terms

1. The application of haircolor to hair that has not been previously colored is called a _____ application.

2. A virgin application indicates that the haircoloring product will be applied to the _____.

3. What is a retouch application? _____
_____

4. What is a line of demarcation? _____
_____

5. Single-process haircoloring is a process that _____ and _____ the hair in a single application.

6. Double-process coloring requires _____ before the _____ color is applied.

7. What is pre-softening and how is it accomplished? _____
_____
_____

8. _____ is the process of coloring some of the hair strands to be lighter than the natural color; _____, _____, and _____ are forms of _____.

9. _____, or _____, is the process of coloring strands or sections of the hair darker than the natural color.

10. Highlights and lowlights can be applied using the _____, _____, or _____ techniques.

TOPIC 7: Haircoloring Product Applications

1. Temporary color rinses are applied at the _____.

2. Temporary color rinses can be used to bring out _____, to temporarily restore _____ hair, to _____ yellow tones, or to tone down _____ hair.

3. List the procedural steps for performing a temporary color rinse application.

   1. _____

   2. _____

   3. _____

   4. _____

   5. _____

4. _____ color products fill the gap between temporary color rinses and permanent haircolor and are _____ colors.

5. Semipermanent tints are considered _____ and do not require the addition of _____.

6. Artificial color added to natural pigment creates a _____ color.

7. Semipermanent tints require a _____ test.

8. Fill in the blanks to complete the steps for performing a semipermanent or demipermanent color application.

   1. Shampoo, rinse, and towel blot hair per _____ directions.

   2. Part hair into _____ sections. Put on gloves. Apply protective cream to hairline.

   3. Apply color in _____ subsections to hair shaft from _____ to ends. Work color through hair until saturated.

   4. Process according to _____ test results and manufacturer's directions. Check color.

   5. After color development, add warm water, _____, and work through hair.

   6. Rinse _____, shampoo, and condition. Remove any stains.

   7. Rinse, towel blot, and _____.

9. Demipermanent color is considered to be _____ color and is applied in the same manner as _____ haircolor.

179

10. Most professional permanent hair coloring is done with the use of _____ penetrating tints that contain _____.

11. Permanent tints are applied on _____ hair.

12. Hair _____ is one of the most important characteristics to consider when choosing hair color tint shades; fill in the blanks to tint darker with the following porosity levels.

    a) normal porosity: _____ than desired color

    b) slightly porous: _____ than desired color

    c) very porous: _____ than desired color

13. To match the natural color of hair and to cover gray, select the color _____ to the natural shade.

14. To brighten or lighten hair color and to cover gray, select a shade _____ than the natural color.

15. To darken the hair and cover gray, select a color _____ than the natural hair color.

16. When tinting lighter than the natural color, use the following steps.

    1. Identify the _____ level.

    2. Identify the _____ level.

    3. _____ the natural level from the desired level.

    4. _____ the level difference to the desired level.

    5. The total is the _____ needed.

17. Fill in the blanks where necessary to complete the steps for performing a single-process permanent color application.

    1. Part dry hair into four sections and put on _____.

    2. Prepare color formula.

    3. Begin in most _____ section.

    4. Part off ¼" subsections and apply color to _____ area; do not apply to the _____.

    5. Process according to strand test results and manufacturer's directions.

    6. Check color development. When desired color is reached, apply remaining product to hair _____ and through to _____.

    7. Lightly wet hair with warm water and lather; massage lather through hair.

    8. Rinse, _____, and condition. Remove stains as necessary.

    9. Rinse, towel blot, and style.

18. When performing a retouch application, apply the tint first to the new hair growth at the _____, _____, and _____ area.

19. Apply tint to new growth in _____ strands and do not _____.

20. Double-process haircoloring begins with hair _____, followed by a _____ or _____.

21. _____ are the mildest form of lightener and lift _____ or _____ levels.

22. Up to _____ activators can be added to _____ lighteners for on-the-scalp applications; up to _____ activators can be added for off-the-scalp processes.

23. _____ lighteners should not be used for retouch applications.

24. Fill in the blanks where necessary to complete the steps for performing a virgin lightening application.

    1. Divide dry hair into four sections.

    2. Apply protective cream around hairline. Put on gloves.

    3. Prepare lightening formula.

    4. _____ in the section where the hair is most resistant.

    5. Part off _____ subsections; apply lightener _____ inch from scalp up to the _____; apply to top and underside of the subsection and place a strip of cotton along the part lines.

    6. _____ comb lightener through the hair.

    7. Process according to strand test results and manufacturer's directions; check lightening action by misting about _____ minutes before required time has elapsed.

    8. Remove cotton from scalp area and apply lightener near the _____ and to porous ends; process until entire hair shaft has reached the desired level.

    9. Rinse, shampoo, and condition; dry the hair and examine scalp for abrasions.

    10. Proceed with _____ application if desired.

25. _____ lightener is usually used for a lightener retouch because it minimizes _____ on the previously lightened hair.

26. _____ have the same chemical ingredients and actions as permanent haircolor products.

27. Toners require a preliminary _____ test 24 hours before the service.

28. A toner is usually applied from the _____ up to the _____.

29. Toner outcomes are dependent on the preliminary _____ treatment.

30. _____ tests are vital to correct double-process applications.

31. Any haircoloring technique that involves the partial lightening or coloring of the hair is called _____ haircoloring.

32. _____ involves lightening strands of hair over various parts of the head.

33. When only the ends of the hair strands are lightened or colored, the process is called

_____.

34. Gray, white, and salt-and-pepper hair having a yellowish cast can be treated with
_____ highlighting shampoos and temporary rinses.

35. Gray hair will usually accept the level of the color applied. Fill in the following table with the recommended formulations for gray hair.

Percentage of Gray	Semipermanent Color Formulation	Permanent Color Formulation
90–100%		
70–90%		
50–70%		
30–50%		
10–30%		

36. _____ can create a color base and help equalize excessive porosity.

37. _____ fillers correct porosity without affecting color and do not deposit a color base.

38. Color fillers are _____ color that will be subdued by the tint.

39. Fillers use _____ colors as pigments and are safe to use without a
_____ test.

40. List some characteristics that damaged hair may exhibit.

    1. _____

    2. _____

    3. _____

    4. _____

    5. _____

    6. _____

    7. _____

41. Returning hair to its natural shade is called a _____.

42. Some over-the-counter hair coloring products are _____ dyes and must be
_____ prior to any other chemical service.

43. The two liquids that are required to perform a test for metallic salts and coating dyes are 20-volume _____ and 28 percent _____.

44. When tested for metallic salts, hair dyed with lead will _____ immediately.

45. When tested for metallic salts, hair treated with copper will start to _____.

46. Hair treated with a coating dye will either _____ or will _____ in spots.

47. Mustaches and beards should never be colored with aniline derivative tints; fill in the blanks to complete the steps for coloring mustaches or beards.

   1. Place client in a _____ position.

   2. Place a clean _____ across the chest.

   3. Wash the _____ with warm, soapy water.

   4. Apply _____ around the hairline of the facial hair.

   5. Apply _____ to the mustache or beard with a moistened cotton-tipped applicator.

   6. Apply _____ to the mustache or beard in same manner.

   7. Wash the _____ with soap and cool water.

   8. Remove any stains with _____.

   9. _____ the mustache or beard as desired.

   10. _____ in the usual manner.

TOPIC 8: Safety Precautions

  1. Fill in the blanks to complete the following haircoloring safety precautions.

   1. Perform a _____ before application of a tint or toner.

   2. _____ the scalp before applying a tint.

   3. _____ apply tint if abrasions are present on the scalp.

   4. Use only _____ materials, tools, and implements.

   5. Always _____ before and after serving a client.

   6. Do not brush the _____ prior to a tint.

   7. Do not apply a tint without _____ directions.

   8. Perform a _____ to determine color results.

   9. Choose tint shade that _____ with the general complexion.

   10. Use an applicator bottle or bowl (plastic or glass) for _____ the tint.

   11. Do not mix tint before _____ for use; discard leftover tint.

   12. If required, use the correct shade of color _____.

13. Make frequent _____ tests until the desired shade is reached.

14. Suggest a _____ treatment for tinted hair.

15. Do not apply tint if _____ or _____ dye is present.

16. Do not apply tint if a patch test is _____.

17. Give a _____ for the correct color shade before applying tint.

18. Do not use an _____ or harsh shampoo for tint removal.

19. Do not use water that is too _____ for removing tint.

20. Protect the client's clothing by proper _____.

21. Do not permit _____ to come in contact with the client's eyes.

22. Do not _____ during a tint retouch.

23. Do not neglect to fill out a tint _____.

24. Do not apply _____ or any material containing hydrogen peroxide directly over dyes known or believed to contain a _____.

25. Wear protective _____.

2. Fill in the blanks to complete the following hair lightening safety precautions.

1. _____ condition of the hair; suggest reconditioning if required.

2. When working with a _____ or _____ lightener, it must be the thickness of whipped cream to avoid dripping or running, causing overlapping.

3. Apply lightener to _____ areas first. Pick up _____ sections when applying lightener.

4. Check strands _____ until the desired shade is reached.

5. After completing the lightener application, check the _____ and _____ any lightener from these areas.

6. Check the towel around the client's neck. Lightener on the towel that is allowed to come in contact with the skin will cause _____.

7. Lightened hair is _____ and requires special care. Use a very _____ shampoo and cool water for rinsing.

8. If a preliminary shampoo is necessary, comb the hair carefully. Avoid irritating the scalp during the _____ or when combing the hair.

9. Work as rapidly as possible when applying the lightener to produce a _____ shade without _____.

10. Never allow lightener to _____; use it immediately.

11. Cap all bottles to avoid _____.

12. Keep a completed _____ of all lightening treatments.

184

Date: _____

Rating: _____

Text Pages 670–702

Chapter 20: Nails and Manicuring

Word Review

Beau's lines	melanonychia	onychomadesis
bed epithelium	nail	onychomycosis
bruised nails	nail bed	onychophagy
cuticle	nail folds	onychorrhexis
eggshell nail	nail grooves	onychosis
eponychium	nail plate	onyx
free edge	nail psoriasis	paronychia
hangnail or agnail	nail pterygium	pincer or trumpet nail
hyponychium	nail unit	plicatured nail
leukonychia spots	onychia	*Pseudomonas aeruginosa*
lunula	onychocryptosis	pyrogenic granuloma
matrix	onycholysis	ridges

TOPIC 1: Introduction

Knowledge of nail structure and manicures provide you with the foundation from which to offer the service or to oversee the procedure as performed by others in your employ.

1. The nail is a horny, translucent plate of _____ that protects the tips of the fingers and toes.

2. Nails are part of the _____ system; they are _____ of the skin.

3. The technical term for nail is _____.

TOPIC 2: Nail Structure

1. The six basic parts of the nail are the nail _____, _____, nail _____, _____ system, specialized _____, and nail _____.

2. Match the following descriptions to the correct part of the nail. Choices may be used more than once.

   _____ most visible and functional portion of the nail   a) nail bed

   _____ living skin that supports the nail plate   b) matrix

   _____ slides along the nail bed as it grows   c) nail plate

   _____ living skin at the base of the nail plate   d) cuticle

   _____ also known as nail root   e) ligaments

   _____ extends to the free edge of the nail   f) nail folds

   _____ layer of skin between free edge and nail plate   g) eponychium

   _____ these form the nail grooves on the sides of the nail   h) hyponychium

   _____ crescent of dead tissue around the nail base

   _____ produces nail plate cells

   _____ attaches the nail bed and matrix to underlying bone

3. Identify the parts of the nail in the following illustration, using the following identifiers: eponychium; matrix; cuticle; nail bed; proximal nail fold; collagen fibers; solehorn; hyponychium; nail plate; distal bed.

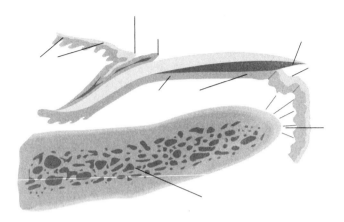

4. Nail growth is influenced by _____ , _____ , and
_____ .

5. The average rate of nail growth in an adult is about _____ "
per _____ .

6. Nails can replace themselves if the _____ remains in good condition.

TOPIC 3: Nail Disorders and Diseases

1. Nail disorders occur as a result of _____ , _____ , or chemical or
nutritional imbalance.

2. If the nail or skin around the nail is infected, inflamed, broken, or swollen, nail
_____ should not be performed.

3. Refer to the textbook to fill in the blanks with the correct name of the nail disorder or disease
described.

   a) _____ technical term for nail deformities or diseases

   b) _____ nails that are thin, whitened, and curved at the free edge

   c) _____ nails with a blood clot under the nail plate

   d) _____ lengthwise ridges on the nail

   e) _____ nails with abnormal color

   f) _____ condition when the cuticle splits around the nail

   g) _____ white spots on the nails

   h) _____ ridges running across the nail

   i) _____ darkening of the nail

   j) _____ ingrown nails

k) _____ deformed bitten nails

l) _____ abnormal splitting or brittle nails

m) _____ skin is stretched by the nail plate

n) _____ fungal infection of the nail

o) _____ inflammation of the matrix with pus and shedding of nail

p) _____ nail separates and falls off from the nail bed

q) _____ loosened nail that does not fall off from the nail bed

r) _____ a bacterial inflammation of tissue around the nail

s) _____ severe inflammation; red tissue in nail plate

t) _____ folded nail

u) _____ curvature of matrix causes curvature of free edge

4. What are five nail disorders or diseases that should not be serviced by a manicurist?
Severe _____ , _____ caused by *Pseudomonas aeruginosa*,
_____ , _____ , or _____ .

TOPIC 4: Introduction to Manicuring

1. List the standard equipment items used in manicuring services.

a) _____

b) _____

c) _____

d) _____

e) _____

f) _____

g) _____

h) _____

2. List the standard implements used in manicuring services.

a) _____

b) _____

c) _____

d) _____

e) _____

f) _____

g) _____

h) _____

3. In your own words, list the steps involved in sanitizing and disinfecting implements effectively.

1. _____

   _____

2. _____

   _____

3. _____

   _____

4. List some commonly used nail cosmetics.

a) _____

b) _____

c) _____

d) _____

e) _____

f) _____

g) _____

h) _____

i) _____

j) _____

k) _____

l) _____

m) _____

n) _____

o) _____

p) _____

5. Polishes are usually applied in four or five coats; list the order in which polish coats are applied.

a) _____

b) _____

c) _____

6. Polish application is started at the _____ of the nail.

7. List the massage movements associated with a hand massage.

1. _____

2. _____

3. _____

4. _____

5. _____

8. After distributing and working in cream or lotion over the client's arm from wrist to elbow, what is the order of applying massage movements in an arm massage?

   1. _____

   2. _____

   3. _____

   4. _____

9. Fill in the blanks to complete the steps of setting up a manicure table.

   1. Wipe the manicure table with an approved _____.

   2. Wrap client cushion in a clean, _____ towel and position in the middle of the table.

   3. Put _____ in bottom of wet sanitizer and fill with disinfectant.

   4. Place cosmetics except _____ on the right side of the table.

   5. Put emery boards and buffers on the _____ side of the table.

   6. Place finger bowl and brush convenient to the _____.

   7. Tape or clip a _____ bag to right side of table.

   8. Place _____ to the left.

   9. Use drawer for _____.

10. What topics should be discussed during the client consultation?

    a) _____

    b) _____

    c) _____

    d) _____

    e) _____

11. Fill in the blanks with the correct name of the following nail shape descriptions.

    a) Nail is shaped straight across: _____ or _____.

    b) Nail is a combination square and oval shape: _____.

    c) Nail has a squoval shape with tapered, rounded corners: _____.

    d) Nail is slightly tapered and extends with a rounded tip: _____.

    e) Nail shape has a longer tapered tip: _____.

12. Most men prefer short _____, _____, or _____ nail shapes.

13. Fill in the blanks where necessary to complete the procedure for a man's manicure.

1. Apply gloves. Set up the manicuring table with the implements and materials.

2. _____. Remove gloves.

3. Greet the client.

4. Wash your hands. _____. Dry hands and nails. Reapply gloves if required by law.

5. Perform client consultation, check for nail _____, and note on client record card.

6. Remove _____ if present.

7. _____ the nails.

8. Soften the cuticles.

9. _____ the nails.

10. Apply cuticle _____.

11. _____ the cuticles.

12. Nip cuticles if client desires and if allowed by state board.

13. Clean under the _____.

14. Repeat steps on other hand.

15. Buff nails if desired.

16. Apply _____ oil.

17. Bevel nails if desired.

18. Apply _____ and _____ hands and arms.

19. _____

20. Apply clear, _____ polish if desired.

21. Schedule next appointment.

22. _____

23. Discard disposables in a closed container.

14. How does a woman's manicure differ from a man's manicure?

_____

_____

15. How is a chair-side manicure performed and what special considerations are required of the manicurist?

_____

_____

_____

_____

Chapter 21: State Board Preparation and Licensing Laws

Word Review

candidate information booklet   practical exam   written exam

TOPIC 1: Introduction

Sitting for your state board examinations is a crucial milestone that marks the beginning of your professional career as you put into practice all that you have learned and mastered.

1. Preparation for state board examinations is under the barbering student's _____.

2. List the factors that will influence how well a candidate performs on state board exams.

    a) _____

    b) _____

    c) _____

    d) _____

    e) _____

3. Most states require written _____ and practical _____ examinations.

TOPIC 2: Preparing for State Board Exams

1. Candidates for written exams must know the _____.

2. List tools and resources that can be used to review the basics for written exams.

    a) _____

    b) _____

    c) _____

    d) _____

    e) _____

3. Always review state barber board _____ to prepare for related questions on written exams.

4. Most written barber exams consist of _____ questions.

5. Oral and/or written directions tell how the questions should be answered and what the _____ are.

6. Some true/false qualifiers to avoid are _____, _____, _____, and _____.

7. When two possible answers in a multiple-choice question are _____, one of them is probably correct.

8. Situational test items provide a _____ from which several different related questions will be asked.

9. Barber law and rules questions on written exams _____ from state to state.

10. Fill in the blanks where necessary to complete a partial list of barber law or rules question items that may be included on a written exam.

   a) Number of _____ members

   b) _____ of the board

   c) Terms of office

   d) Exemptions and _____

   e) Examination _____

   f) Types of licenses

   g) License _____

   h) License _____ dates

   i) Fees and penalties

   j) Minimum _____ for a barbershop

   k) Continuing education _____

   l) Prohibited acts

   m) Qualifications for _____

11. Basic skills and procedures usually evaluated during practical exams include _____, _____, _____, _____, and sometimes a _____ service.

12. Standard testing protocol usually requires candidates to demonstrate competence with the _____, _____, _____, and _____ and to use _____ precautions, proper _____, and safe _____ handling.

13. Practical exams are the best way to evaluate a person's _____ in barbering techniques.

14. Basic preparation for practical exams should always include _____ on the _____ that will be taken to the examination.

15. Performance confidence starts with familiarity of the model's hair _____ and the _____ to be performed.

192

16. Many states require a _____ haircut for the practical examination.

17. Fill in the blanks to complete the suggestions for practical exam practice.

   a) Set up the _____ as if at the _____ examinations.

   b) Make sure that all tools and implements are _____ and in good _____.

   c) Practice all _____ procedures, including _____.

   d) _____ yourself.

   e) Request _____ from instructors and models.

   f) Be clear about what examiners will check and look for in the _____ of procedures.

   g) Read your state board _____ to find specific exam information.

   h) Review the _____ booklet for specifics about practical testing.

18. Exam candidates should confirm the test _____, _____, and _____ arrangements with their model several _____ before the test date.

19. If the test site is out of town, candidates should consider arriving the day _____ the exams.

20. Create a checklist of the _____, _____, and _____ needed for practical exams; make sure tools are cleaned and _____.

21. Consult _____ materials for required tools and procedures.

22. Dress comfortably but _____ for the exams; _____ wear a name tag or school insignia.

TOPIC 3: State Barber Board Rules and Regulations

1. The basic goal and function of state barber boards is to protect the _____, _____, and _____ of the _____ as it relates to the practice of _____.

2. Fill in the blanks to complete the following statements related to state barber boards.

   a) The government body that is responsible for the efficient and orderly administration of barbering rules and regulations is the _____.

   b) The authority to conduct _____ rests with the state barber board.

   c) Additional authority that is given to the state barber board in order to properly administer barber license law is the power to _____.

   d) The primary objective of the barber license law is to _____ the health, safety, and welfare of the public.

e) The _____ of the state appoints barber board members.

f) The _____ confirms the appointment of barber board members.

g) The state barber board regulates _____, _____,
_____, _____, _____, and
_____.

h) The objective of barber license examinations is to evaluate a license applicant's
_____.

i) State Barber Board rules and regulations _____ be used to limit the number of licenses or licensees.

j) An important personal requirement for a barber license applicant is to be of good
_____.

k) Barbers may be forbidden to perform services on clients when the barber is suffering from a
_____.

l) State barber boards may discipline a barber by _____ or
_____ of the barber's license.

m) Licensed barbers are protected by the laws of the state against _____ action by the state barber board.

n) Licensed barbers must be granted a _____ before the state barber board can take action to _____ or _____ a license.

o) A licensee who violates the provisions of the barber license law can be cited for
_____.

p) Persons who act as a barber without obtaining a license are guilty of _____ in a/an _____ manner.

q) A barber who has his license suspended or revoked has the _____ to the courts.

r) A person convicted of violating any of the provisions of the license law is guilty of a
_____.

s) The purpose of periodic inspections of barbershops is to ascertain compliance with
_____ regulations and _____ compliance.

t) A licensee who willfully fails to display a _____ or _____
is guilty of a _____ of the barber law.

u) Barber law requires that suspended or revoked licenses must be surrendered to the
_____.

v) The state barber board may suspend or revoke the license of a licensee who is guilty of
_____.

w) The barbershop _____ is responsible for posting _____, barber law, and the state board rules and regulations in the barbershop.

x) The state barber board may suspend or revoke the license of a licensee who is guilty of
_____.

y) An apprentice practices barbering under the _____ and direct supervision of a
_____ barber.

z) Generally speaking, persons who are legally _____ from barber law provisions
while working within the provisions of their own professions are medical personnel, military
personnel, and cosmetologists.

Chapter 22: The Job Search

Word Review

booth renter	employee status	portfolio
commission	model release form	résumé
cover letter		

TOPIC 1: Introduction

This chapter has been provided to assist you in your search for employment in the barbering field.

1. It appears the need for barbers and barbershops has been on a steady increase since the

    _____ .

2. Since the 1970s, _____ have offered services to the male haircutting market.

3. Fill in the blanks to complete some of the needs of the barbering profession.

    a) _____ designed to meet expectation and service requirements for a variety of male preferences

    b) Barbers to pass along their skills and professional _____ to others as teachers, _____ members, and association leaders

    c) Skilled artisans to participate in _____ at hair and trade shows

    d) _____ to protect the barbering profession and its future

    e) New young barbers to replace _____ practitioners

TOPIC 2: Preparing for Employment

1. Whether or not a student barber is allowed to work in a barbershop while training depends on the laws, rules, and regulations of the _____ .

2. Fill in the blanks to complete the benefits student barbers may achieve by participating in the operations of a barbershop or salon while still in training.

    a) Exposure to the _____ , _____ , and services of the shop

    b) Understanding of _____ tasks and responsibilities of shop personnel

    c) Experience in _____ with clients and coworkers

    d) Experience in perfecting _____ skills

    e) _____ of advanced services, techniques, and skills

    f) Familiarity with shop _____ and _____

g) _____ to lay the foundation for future _____

h) _____ gain

3. What questions might you ask yourself when considering where to work in the future?

a) _____

b) _____

c) _____

4. Identify one action that can help student barbers determine where they would like to work.

_____

5. List some practical applications used to prepare for employment.

a) _____

b) _____

c) _____

d) _____

e) _____

6. In your own words, list some guidelines for goal setting.

a) _____

b) _____

c) _____

d) _____

e) _____

7. List some industry-related opportunities that can help prepare barbering students for employment.

a) _____

b) _____

c) _____

d) _____

8. Match the following descriptions of personal characteristics with the correct term. Choices may be used more than once.

_____ a compass that guides people in what they say and do

_____ the drive necessary to take action to achieve a goal

_____ a commitment to delivering quality service

_____ one of a person's strongest marketing tools

_____ demonstrates passion for what one is doing

_____ accounts for about 80 percent of a person's success

_____ internally or externally driven

_____ accounts for about 20 percent of a person's success

_____ demonstrated by a belief that work is good

_____ a strong commitment to a code of morals and values

a) motivation

b) integrity

c) technical skills

d) communication and people skills

e) strong work ethic

f) enthusiasm

g) attitude

9. The way a barber is paid for services performed in the barbershop depends primarily on the barber's _____ classification.

10. Employment status classifications for barbers include _____, _____, and _____.

11. Independent contractors and booth renters are classified as _____ workers.

12. Employees may be paid on a salary, _____, or salary-plus-commission basis.

13. Employers are responsible for withholding income tax and _____, paying a portion of an employee's social security tax, _____ taxes, and issuing a Form W-2, *Wage and Tax Statement*.

14. Employees are responsible for reporting _____ and commissions, and filing personal income tax returns.

15. Independent contractors may rent chair or work for a percentage but must apply for a _____ number. They must also provide _____ insurance, be responsible for all taxes, and have a _____ with the owner to _____ their independent contractor status.

16. In a booth rental situation, the fees brought in from services are basically the barber's after paying for the _____ and _____.

17. Booth renters assume almost all the responsibilities of small business ownership and must have a rental _____ with the shop owner.

18. The booth renter's clientele should be large enough to cover _____ and pay the barber a salary.

19. Independent contractors and employees may be paid on a _____, commission, or salary-plus-commission basis.

20. A written summary of one's education, work experience, and achievements is called a
_____.

21. Fill in the blanks to develop a rough draft of a resume based on your current experience and accomplishments.

```
                        Name
                        Address
                        Phone
                        Email


        Objective:


        Education:


        Experience:


        Accomplishments:


        Honors and Awards:

```

22. A _____ is used to introduce the job applicant to the employer and to reference the position being sought.

23. Cover letters can be used to expand on _____ mentioned in the resume.

24. A collection of photographs depicting the barber's ability to provide haircare services is called a _____.

25. A portfolio should contain _____ and _____ photos of the barber's _____ work.

26. The client's or model's _____ must be gained before photographing the barber's work.

27. Clients and models should sign a _____ or _____.

28. List some resources a barber student can use to find local barbershops for his or her job search.

a) _____

b) _____

c) _____

d) _____

e) _____

f) _____

g) _____

h) _____

29. List three reasons why a student barber might engage in field research.

1. _____

2. _____

3. _____

30. Before visiting a shop or salon, student barbers should contact the shop owner by

_____ .

31. Put networking on a _____ level by mentioning mutual contacts during the telephone conversation.

32. _____ can lead to jobs not advertised in the newspaper.

33. After passing state board examinations, graduate barbers should contact prospective employers by sending them a resume with a _____ that requests an _____ .

34. Job applicants should offer to bring a _____ to demonstrate technical skills.

35. It is a standard practice in barbering for an employer to require a job applicant to perform a _____ or other service on a _____ as part of the interview process.

TOPIC 3: The Employment Interview

1. One way to prepare for the interview is have all _____ in one place.

2. Support materials include identification, _____ , résumé, portfolio, and the _____ if available.

3. Job applicants should be prepared to answer questions about their _____ , _____ , and _____ relations skills.

4. Job applicants should be prepared with _____ they would like to have answered before making the decision to work in the barbershop.

5. Job applicants should " _____ for success."

6. List some behaviors that should be demonstrated during the interview.

a) _____

b) _____

c) _____

d) _____

e) _____

f) _____

g) _____

h) _____

7. List some questions a job applicant might ask of the interviewer.

   a) _____

   b) _____

   c) _____

   d) _____

   e) _____

8. List some other factors that an applicant needs to consider before accepting a position.

   a) _____

   b) _____

   c) _____

   d) _____

   e) _____

   f) _____

   g) _____

   h) _____

   i) _____

9. Fill in the blank to complete the question topics that may not be asked on an employment application or during an interview.

   a) _____ , religion, and _____ origin

   b) _____ status

   c) _____ or physical traits

   d) _____ status

   e) height and _____

   f) _____ record

   g) _____

10. Questions that may be asked in an interview are those related to _____ , _____ , or _____ if necessary to verify minimum requirements for the job.

Chapter 23: Barbershop Management

Word Review

booth renter	employee	sole proprietor
business plan	franchise ownership	S corporation
capital	independent contractor	target market
corporation	limited liability company	
demographics	partnership	

TOPIC 1: Introduction

1. Business ownership requires the knowledge and application of business principles, _____ and business law, financial management, salesmanship, human relations skills, and operational management expertise.

2. Barbershop ownership and daily management involve the direct control and coordination of all _____ .

TOPIC 2: Self-employment and Business Ownership

1. Business ownership requires commitment and follow-through. Be prepared to _____ the business idea before making _____ or signing contracts.

2. Business _____ involves planning, decision making, financial obligations, compliance, and many other details of business operations. _____ is concerned with production and daily operations as applied to the business and the people working in it.

3. In most barbershops, the owner is one of the _____ .

4. Fill in the blanks to complete the basic tasks that need to be done before opening a barbershop.

    1. Determine the type of _____ .

    2. Review tax laws to help determine worker _____ .

    3. Retain a _____ and an accountant.

    4. Determine the _____ to be offered and the _____ to be reached.

    5. Determine the type of shop _____ desired.

    6. Find a suitable _____ and research costs.

    7. Create a _____ .

    8. Arrange for financing or _____ investment.

9. Plan and research equipment, fixtures, and furnishings _____.

10. Establish a _____-keeping system.

11. Establish shop policies, _____, and protocols.

12. Arrange for advertising and _____.

13. _____, hire, and train employees.

14. Design a plan to establish good _____ within the community.

5. Identify six types of business structures appropriate for barbershop ownership.

a) _____

b) _____

c) _____

d) _____

e) _____

f) _____

6. Match each of the following business models with its appropriate characteristic or feature.

_____ two or more individuals share ownership   a) sole proprietorship

_____ available to individuals or groups   b) partnership

_____ requires formal records like a corporation   c) corporation

_____ owner responsible for all profits and losses   d) limited liability company

_____ individuals must meet established criteria   e) subchapter's corporation

_____ stockholders not legally responsible for losses   f) franchise

TOPIC 3: Employment Classifications

1. Worker classifications are used to determine the party or entity that has the responsibility to pay _____.

2. As a barbershop owner, you will have to decide if other barbers in the shop will work as employees, _____, or booth renters.

3. Employees may be paid on a _____, commission, or salary-plus-commission basis.

4. Employers are responsible for providing _____ guidelines for employees; withholding income, Medicare, unemployment, and employee _____ taxes; and providing _____ forms for all employees.

5. Employers need to keep records that document employees' monthly _____ over $20.00 and _____ paid for product sales.

6. Independent contractors may rent a chair or work for a _____ of service sales.

7. Independent contractors must have their own business insurance and _____ identification number. They are responsible for their own income and _____ taxes.

8. To be classified as an independent contractor there must be a _____ agreement drawn up between the owner and the contractor.

9. Independent contractors should receive a _____ form from the owner at the end of the tax year.

10. In a _____ arrangement, the shop owner provides space to be leased and the barber operates a _____ within the confines of the shop.

11. The IRS tax designation for a booth renter is booth renter or independent _____, not _____.

12. Booth renters need to have a _____ contract with the shop owner.

13. Booth renters are solely responsible for their own taxes, licenses, insurance, clientele, supplies, record keeping, accounting, and so forth, and must provide the shop owner with a _____ form at the end of the tax year for the _____ paid.

TOPIC 4: Purchasing an Established Barbershop

1. An established barbershop is in operation when it is put on the market for sale and has a solid, repeat _____ base.

2. Fill in the blanks to complete the questions that should be asked and investigated before a sales agreement is signed.

   a) Is the mortgage, bill of sale, or lease _____ without any liens against it?

   b) Are there any _____ in the payment of debts?

   c) Are all state, federal, property, and Social Security taxes, and other obligations paid and _____?

   d) Are there lease or current tenant _____ that have to be addressed?

3. Fill in the blanks to complete some items that a purchase agreement should include.

   a) _____ purchase and sale agreement with contact information of both parties

   b) A complete and _____ statement of inventory indicating the value of each item

   c) Use of the shop's _____ and reputation for a definite amount of time (if desired)

   d) Disclosure of the business's accounts, tax information, and _____ statements

   e) Information about the shop's clientele regarding their purchasing and _____ habits

   f) A _____ or non-compete clause prohibiting the seller from competing with the new owner within a specified distance from the present location.

204

TOPIC 5: Establishing a Barbershop

1. Services to be offered and targeted markets help to determine a barbershop's potential for _____.

2. A barbershop should be clean, comfortable, _____, and appealing.

3. Visibility, parking, signage, competition, and public transportation access are some features associated with a good _____.

4. Marketing and advertising efforts should be directed toward the _____ market or audience.

5. Local ordinances should be checked to make certain the area is _____ for the operation of a barbershop.

6. A _____ protects the shop owner against unexpected increases in rent, protects the right of continued occupancy, and sets forth the rights and obligations of the _____ and tenant.

7. An _____ should review the lease to ensure it contains all the provisions and agreements made between the landlord and the tenant.

8. Fill in the blanks to complete some possible inclusions in a lease agreement.

   a) An exemption allowing for _____ of certain fixtures or structures unnecessary to the barbershop without _____ of the lease

   b) All agreements concerning _____, _____, plumbing, painting, fixtures, and electrical installations

   c) An _____ that makes provision for the lessee to assign the lease to another person in case a partnership develops or a new owner takes over the business

9. What is a business plan?

   _____

   _____

10. Business plans should be developed from information gathered during _____.

11. Fill in the blanks to complete some elements of a business plan.

    a) A general description of the business and the _____ it will provide

    b) The number of personnel to be hired, their _____ or _____ contributions, and other benefits

    c) An _____ plan

    d) A _____ plan including a profit and loss statement

    e) A detailed listing of _____ costs

12. A good business plan provides an accurate _____ of the money needed to _____ and _____ the business.

13. Investment money used to cover expenses is called _____.

14. A new barbershop should have sufficient capital to cover expenses for _____.

15. The number one reason for business failure is _____.

16. Barbershops must comply with local, state, and federal _____ and
    _____.

17. _____ regulations may govern building codes, zoning laws, and occupational or
    business licenses.

18. _____ laws cover sales taxes, professional and business licenses, and workers'
    compensation.

19. _____ and _____ governments govern income tax laws.

20. _____ law governs income tax, social security, unemployment insurance,
    cosmetics and luxury tax payments, and OSHA safety and health standards.

21. Some _____ used in business establishments include malpractice, premises
    liability, fire, burglary and theft, and business interruption coverage.

22. Barbershops should be designed to achieve maximum _____ and economy
    of space.

23. Fill in the blanks to complete the factors that should be planned for in the design of the
    barbershop.

    a) Maximum efficiency of _____

    b) Adequate _____ space

    c) Adequate space for each piece of _____

    d) Quality _____

    e) _____, furniture, and equipment chosen for cost, _____,
       utility, and appearance

    f) _____ and décor that is restful and pleasing to the eye

    g) Adequate _____ for clients and employees

    h) _____-access facilities and doors

    i) Good _____ and sufficient _____ for services

    j) Proper _____, air conditioning, and heating

    k) Sufficient electrical _____, and _____ to adequately service
       all equipment

    l) Adequate _____ areas

    m) An attractive _____ or waiting area

    n) Sufficient _____ areas

206

24. Sanitation and _____ procedures must be strictly enforced at all times.

25. Always consult _____ regulations when designing the barbershop.

26. _____ includes all activities that attract attention to the barbershop.

TOPIC 6: Barbershop Ownership Exercise

1. You have decided to open your own barbershop. What does it look like?

_____
_____
_____
_____
_____
_____
_____
_____
_____
_____

2. Describe the location.

_____
_____
_____
_____
_____
_____
_____
_____
_____
_____

3. What is the name of your barbershop?

_____

4. Who is your target clientele?

_____
_____

5. How do you plan to reach your target market?

_____
_____
_____
_____
_____
_____
_____
_____

6. What types of services do you plan to offer?

_____

_____

7. Where will your start-up costs come from?

_____

_____

8. How will you maintain the shop and your personal expenses until the shop is successful?

_____

_____

9. Draw a picture of your business sign in the space provided.

10. Draw a floor plan of your barbershop in the space provided.

TOPIC 7: The Barbershop

1. The barbershop should be clean, comfortable, _____, and appealing.

2. List some of the features associated with a good location.

    a) _____

    b) _____

    c) _____

    d) _____

    e) _____

    f) _____

    g) _____

3. List some of the site characteristics that should be judged when deciding on the space.

    a) _____

    b) _____

    c) _____

    d) _____

    e) _____

    f) _____

    g) _____

    h) _____

    i) _____

4. List some advertising venues that may be used to promote the barbershop.

    a) _____

    b) _____

    c) _____

    d) _____

    e) _____

    f) _____

    g) _____

    h) _____

    i) _____

    j) _____

    k) _____

l) _____

m) _____

n) _____

o) _____

5. _____ can be designed into all print on online advertising.

6. _____ and _____ service encourages clients to return and recommend the shop to others.

7. The best form of advertising is a _____ and _____ client.

8. Fill in the blanks to complete some actions that can help protect the shop from fire, theft, or lawsuits.

   a) Keep the premises securely _____.

   b) Follow _____ precautions to prevent fire, injury, and lawsuits.

   c) Purchase liability, _____, fire, and burglary insurance.

   d) Never violate _____, law by attempting to diagnose, treat, or cure disease. Refer client to a physician.

   e) Become thoroughly familiar with barbering laws and _____ codes.

   f) Keep _____ of workers, salaries, length of employment, and social security numbers for state and federal laws affecting employees.

   g) Maintain a _____ notebook.

9. List the qualities required for successful business operation.

   a) _____

   b) _____

   c) _____

   d) _____

   e) _____

10. Besides efficient and effective management, what other factors does the success of a business depend on?

   a) _____

   b) _____

   c) _____

   d) _____

   e) _____

   f) _____

11. Fill in the blanks to complete some contributing causes of business failures.

    a) _____ in dealing with the public and employees

    b) Insufficient capital to _____ the business until established

    c) Poor _____

    d) High cost of _____

    e) Lack of proper basic _____

    f) _____ bookkeeping methods

    g) _____ of the business

    h) Lack of _____ personnel

12. _____ means keeping an accurate record of all income and expenses.

13. _____ is the money generated from services and retail sales.

14. _____ are the cost of doing business.

15. An _____ helps to keep records accurate and processed in a timely manner.

16. Proper _____ are necessary to meet the requirements of local, state, and federal laws regarding taxes and employees. Proper records are also required for efficient _____; determining _____, expenses, profit, and loss; assessing the _____ of the business; and for arranging a bank loan.

17. One simple method of bookkeeping for the barbershop is to maintain a daily account of the _____ and _____ of the shop.

18. The difference between total income and total expense is called _____.

19. A profit occurs when _____ is greater than the _____; a loss occurs when _____ are greater than the _____.

20. An _____ helps to keep expenditures on track.

21. A summary sheet helps the business owner to make _____ with other years, to detect changes in demand for different _____, and to _____ expenses and waste.

22. Daily sales slips, appointment books, and petty cash receipts should be kept for at least _____.

23. Payroll records, cancelled checks, and monthly and yearly records are usually held for _____.

24. An inventory system can help prevent _____ or _____ of supplies.

25. Service records are also called _____.

TOPIC 8: Operating a Successful Barbershop

1. One of the keys to a prosperous barbershop is to _____.

2. What personal characteristics should be considered when interviewing a prospective employee?

   a) _____

   b) _____

   c) _____

   d) _____

   e) _____

3. A checklist can be used to _____ job applicants in categories important to shop success.

4. _____ should be used to measure or evaluate a job applicant.

5. Fill in the blanks to complete some general guidelines used for effective personnel management.

   a) Be _____ with employees

   b) Expect the _____

   c) Be a _____

   d) _____ information

   e) Follow the _____

6. The best business environment is one in which everyone feels _____, enjoys _____ hard, and strives to provide _____ to the customers.

7. The location of the shop and the type of clientele it serves usually guides the _____ of services.

8. _____ should be posted where clients will see them.

9. The _____ area is the first area of the shop that clients see; it should be attractive, appealing, and comfortable.

10. Appointments are booked in terms of the amount of _____ it takes to do the service.

11. Depending on the size of the shop and the owner's preferences, appointments may be booked by the _____ or the _____.

12. The majority of barbershop business is handled over the _____.

13. Fill in the blanks where necessary to list some ways telephones are used on a daily basis in the barbershop.

    a) Make or change _____

    b) Seek new business

    c) _____ clients of their appointments

212

d) Answer questions and render friendly service

e) Handle _____ to the client's satisfaction

f) Receive _____

g) _____ equipment and supplies

h) Provide _____ to clients

i) Provide shop _____

j) Determine who is on staff that day

14. The shop's _____ should be displayed on stationery, advertising circulars, and business cards.

15. _____ should be available in the waiting area and at each station.

16. Fill in the blanks to complete the following telephone etiquette reminders:

a) Answer all calls as _____ as possible.

b) Express an interested and helpful _____.

c) Identify _____ and the _____ when making or receiving a call.

d) Be _____.

e) Inquire as to the caller's name by saying, _____

f) Address people by their appropriate _____ and _____.

g) Use _____ expressions.

h) Avoid making side remarks or speaking to _____ during a call.

i) Let the _____ end the conversation.

j) Do not hang up _____ at the end of a call.

17. A good telephone personality includes _____ speech, _____ speech patterns, and a pleasing _____ of voice.

18. All greetings and automated messages should be _____ appropriate with no _____ music, language, or _____.

19. When booking a client appointment, record the _____, _____, and requested _____.

20. Mark out the appropriate _____ for the requested service on the appointment book.

21. What are some things you can do if the requested barber is not available for the client?

_____

_____

22. When handling complaints, respond with _____, _____, and _____.

TOPIC 9: Selling in the Barbershop

1. Revenue in the barbershop is derived from the performance of _____ and the sale of _____ .

2. To close a sale, the client must perceive the service or product as _____ .

3. A _____ -sell approach should never be used; conversely, the sales approach should be subtle, friendly, honest, and _____ .

4. The barber's _____ can influence and arouse a client's interest in other styling and grooming services.

5. In order to sell additional services to clients, the barber must be _____ of each service, know _____ , and be able to _____ to be derived from it.

6. List some services that might be suggested to a client:

   a) _____

   b) _____

   c) _____

   d) _____

   e) _____

   f) _____

   g) _____

   h) _____

   i) _____

7. _____ products sold in the barbershop should be used during _____ performed in the shop.

8. List some standard grooming supplies that a barbershop might retail to its customers:

   a) _____

   b) _____

   c) _____

   d) _____

   e) _____

   f) _____

   g) _____

   h) _____

   i) _____

Notes

Notes